MAKING SENSE

of the ECG

CASES FOR
SELF-ASSESSMENT

MAKING SENSE

of the ECG

**CASES FOR
SELF-ASSESSMENT**

Andrew R. Houghton
MA(Oxon) DM FRCP(Lond) FRCP(Glasg)
Consultant Cardiologist
Grantham and District Hospital
Grantham, UK
and
Visiting Fellow
University of Lincoln
Lincoln, UK

David Gray
DM MPH BMedSci FRCP(Lond) FRIPH
Reader in Medicine and Honorary
Consultant Physician
Department of Cardiovascular Medicine
University Hospital, Queen's Medical Centre,
Nottingham, UK

**HODDER
ARNOLD**
AN HACHETTE UK COMPANY

First published in Great Britain in 2009 by
Hodder Arnold, an imprint of Hodder Education, an Hachette UK Company,
338 Euston Road, London NW1 3BH

http://www.hoddereducation.com

*Hachette UK's policy is to use papers that are natural, renewable and recyclable
products and made from wood grown in sustainable forests. The logging and
manufacturing processes are expected to conform to the environmental regulations
of the country of origin.*

Whilst the advice and information in this book are believed to be true and accurate at
the date of going to press, neither the authors nor the publisher can accept any legal
responsibility or liability for any errors or omissions that may be made. In particular
(but without limiting the generality of the preceding disclaimer) every effort has been
made to check drug dosages; however it is still possible that errors have been missed.
Furthermore, dosage schedules are constantly being revised and new side-effects
recognized. For these reasons the reader is strongly urged to consult the drug
companies' printed instructions before administering any of the drugs recommended
in this book.

British Library Cataloguing in Publication Data
A catalogue record for this book is available from the British Library

Library of Congress Cataloging-in-Publication Data
A catalog record for this book is available from the Library of Congress

ISBN   978 0 340 946 893

1 2 3 4 5 6 7 8 9 10

Commissioning Editor:	Sara Purdy
Project Editor:	Jane Tod and Eva Senior
Production Controller:	Andre Sim and Karen Tate
Cover Designer:	Amina Dudhia
Indexer:	Lisa Footitt

Typeset in 10/11 Chaparra MM 250 LT by Macmillan Publishing Solutions
(www.macmillansolutions.com)

Printed and bound in India

What do you think about this book? Or any other Hodder Arnold title?
Please visit our website: www.hoddereducation.com

To Kathryn and Caroline

Contents

Preface

If you have already read our book *Making Sense of the ECG* you may now be keen to put your knowledge to the test. In this companion volume, *Making Sense of the ECG: Cases for Self-Assessment*, you can test your skills in ECG interpretation with 70 individual clinical cases.

This book is simple to use. Each of the 70 cases begins with an ECG, an illustrative clinical scenario (to place the ECG in an appropriate context), and a number of questions. On turning the page, you will find the answers to the questions together with a detailed analysis of the ECG. This is followed by a general commentary on the ECG and the clinical case, and suggestions for further reading. The ECG cases are presented in order of increasing difficulty and we are certain that, whatever your experience in ECG interpretation, you will find cases to challenge your skills.

We are grateful to everyone who has taken the time to comment on the cases and to help us acquire ECGs for this book. Finally, we would like to thank all of the staff at Hodder Arnold who have contributed to the success of the *Making Sense of the ECG* books.

Andrew R. Houghton
David Gray
2009

Note: Every time *Making Sense of the ECG* is referred to in Further reading sections, this is a cross-reference to the companion book: Houghton AR and Gray D (2008). *Making Sense of the ECG, Third Edition*, London: Hodder Arnold.

Acknowledgements

We would like to thank everyone who gave us suggestions and constructive criticism while we prepared *Making Sense of the ECG: Cases for Self-Assessment*. We are particularly grateful to the following for their comments on the text and for assisting us in acquiring the ECGs for this book:

Mookhter Ajij
Denise Archer
Stephanie Baker
Michael Bamber
Andrea Charman
Matthew Donnelly
Lawrence Green
Mahesh Harishchandra
Daniel Law
Diane Lunn

Cara Mercer
Emma Murphy
Vicky Nelmes
Claire Poole
Jane Robinson
Catherine Scott
Penelope R. Sensky
Nimit Shah
Upul Wijayawardhana
Bernadette Williamson

We are grateful to the BMJ Publishing Group for their permission to reproduce ECGs from their publications in Cases 37, 46, 55, 59, 63 and 68.

Finally, we would also like to express our gratitude to everyone at Hodder Arnold for their guidance and support.

Normal values

Full blood count (FBC)

Hb	13.5–16.9 g/dL (male); 11.5–14.8 g/dL (female)
White cell count (WCC)	4.5–13.0 $\times$ 10^9/L
Platelets	150–400 $\times$ 10^9/L

Urea and electrolytes (U&E)

Na	136–145 mmol/L
K	3.5–5.1 mmol/L
Urea	3.2–7.4 mmol/L (male); 2.5–6.7 mmol/L (female)
Creatinine	53–115 mmol/L

CASE 1

Clinical scenario

Male, aged 28 years.

Presenting complaint
Asymptomatic fitness instructor. This screening ECG was performed at a 'well man' medical check-up.

History of presenting complaint
Nil – the patient is asymptomatic.

Past medical history
Appendicectomy (aged 17 years).

Examination
Athletic build.
Pulse: 50 bpm, regular.
Blood pressure: 128/80.
JVP: not elevated.
Heart sounds: normal.
Chest auscultation: unremarkable.
No peripheral oedema.
Old appendicectomy scar noted in right iliac fossa.

Investigations
FBC: Hb 14.8, WCC 6.2, platelets 229.
U&E: Na 140, K 4.4, urea 3.7, creatinine 78.
Thyroid function: normal.
Chest X-ray: normal heart size, clear lung fields.

Questions

1 What does this ECG show?
2 How did you calculate the heart rate?
3 Is the heart rate normal?
4 Is any further action required?

ECG analysis

Rate	50 bpm
Rhythm	Sinus bradycardia
QRS axis	Normal (+42°)
P waves	Normal
PR interval	Normal (160 ms)
QRS duration	Normal (76 ms)
T waves	Normal
QTc interval	Normal (407 ms)

Additional comments

There is a very slight variation in heart rate on the ECG – the distance between consecutive QRS complexes (the R-R interval) varies slightly. This is not unusual, and results from a slight variation in heart rate with respiration.

Answers

1 This ECG shows mild sinus bradycardia, but is otherwise normal.

2 There are two ways to calculate heart rate:
• At a standard paper speed of 25 mm/s, there will be 300 large squares for every minute of ECG recording.

You can therefore count the number of large squares between two consecutive QRS complexes – in this example, there are 6 – and then divide this number into 300 (i.e. 300/6). This gives a heart rate of 50 bpm. This method is best used when the rhythm is regular.

• Alternatively, you can count the total number of QRS complexes along a strip 30 large squares in length. A strip of 30 large squares is equivalent to 6 s of recording (at a paper speed of 25 mm/s). You can therefore count the number of QRS complexes in 30 large squares, and then multiply this number by 10 to give the number of QRS complexes per minute This method is particularly useful for irregular rhythms such as atrial fibrillation.

3 Generally speaking, bradycardia is defined as a heart rate below 60 bpm. However, it is always important to assess clinical data in the context of the patient. This is a young patient, with an athletic background, and so a relatively slow resting heart rate is not unusual. In this clinical context, the mild sinus bradycardia is not of concern.

4 No – the patient can be reassured that the ECG is normal.

Commentary

● One of the most important principles of ECG interpretation, and indeed in interpreting any test result, is to place things in their clinical context. Although the 'normal range' for the heart rate in sinus rhythm is 60–100 bpm, a rate between 50–60 bpm is seldom of any significance or clinical consequence. If a patient is athletic, it is not unusual to have a mild resting bradycardia and it is important not to diagnose this as pathological.

● Whenever you interpret an ECG, it is important to begin by asking 'How is the patient?' This will give you the clinical context you require to make a correct assessment. Similarly, if you make an ECG recording, it is good practice to make a note of the clinical context at the top of the ECG, along with the patient's identification

details and the date/time of the recording. This can take the form of a brief sentence to say 'Patient complaining of palpitations', or 'Patient experiencing 6/10 chest tightness', or just 'Routine ECG – patient asymptomatic'. This makes it much easier for you – and for others – to interpret the ECG when it is reviewed later on.

● A mild sinus bradycardia can also be the result of drug treatment (particularly beta blockers, digoxin or rate-limiting calcium channel blockers, such as verapamil). Don't forget about beta blocking eye drops, which can have systemic effects.

● The T wave inversion seen in lead aVR and in lead V_1 is a normal finding.

Further reading

Making Sense of the ECG: Heart rate, p 19; Sinus rhythm, p 29; Sinus bradycardia, p 31.

CASE 2

Speed: 25 mm/s   Limb: 10 mm/mV   Chest: 10 mm/mV

Clinical scenario

Male, aged 27 years.

Presenting complaint

No cardiac symptoms but aware he has an 'abnormal ECG'.

History of presenting complaint

Patient had been scheduled for knee surgery and was seen by a nurse in the surgical preoperative assessment clinic. The nurse reported a slightly irregular pulse and requested an ECG. Subsequently the patient was referred to the cardiology clinic for a preoperative cardiac opinion.

Past medical history

Nil of note.

Examination

Pulse: 60 bpm, slightly irregular.
Blood pressure: 126/88.
JVP: not elevated.
Heart sounds: normal.
Chest auscultation: unremarkable.
No peripheral oedema.

Investigations

FBC: Hb 16.5, WCC 4.3, platelets 353.
U&E: Na 140, K 4.5, urea 4.4, creatinine 98.
Thyroid function: normal.
Chest X-ray: normal heart size, clear lung fields.

Questions

1 What does this ECG show?
2 What is the mechanism of this?
3 What is the likely cause?
4 What are the key issues in managing this patient?

ECG analysis

Rate	60 bpm
Rhythm	Sinus arrhythmia
QRS axis	Normal (+43°)
P waves	Normal
PR interval	Normal (160 ms)
QRS duration	Normal (100 ms)
T waves	Normal
QTc interval	Normal (400 ms)

Answers

1 Every P wave is followed by a normal QRS complex, but the heart rate varies. Observation of the patient confirms that this coincides with respiration, with the heart rate increasing on inspiration and decreasing on expiration. This is **sinus arrhythmia**.

2 There is variation in the heart rate in response to respiration, increasing reflexly during inspiration (due to increased venous return to the heart) and decreasing during expiration.

3 This is a normal physiological response. The exact mechanism of sinus arrhythmia has been the subject of investigation and debate for many years. There is some evidence that the respiratory variation in heart rate is mediated via carotid baroreceptors and/or cardio-pulmonary receptors. Others suggest a central mechanism. (Heart rate is normally controlled by centres in the medulla oblongata. One centre, the nucleus ambiguus, provides parasympathetic input to the heart via the vagus nerve, affecting the sinoatrial node. Inspiration signals the nucleus accumbens to inhibit the vagus nerve, increasing heart rate, while expiration increases vagal activity and reduces heart rate.)

4 No action is needed. Reassure the patient (and the pre-assessment clinic staff) that sinus arrhythmia is a normal finding.

Commentary

● Sinus arrhythmia is of no pathological consequence. Sinus arrhythmia is most often seen in the young and much less commonly in those over the age of 40 years.

● Normally, the heart rate in sinus rhythm changes very little at rest. In sinus arrhythmia, the slight variation in cycling usually exceeds 120 ms between the longest and the shortest cycle (cycle length is equal to the interval between successive R waves, the RR interval).

● Sinus arrhythmia may be aggravated by any factor that increases vagal tone.

Further reading

Making Sense of the ECG: Sinus arrhythmia, p 34; Irregular cardiac rhythms, p 68.

Piepoli M, Sleight P, Leuzzi, S, *et al.* Origin of respiratory sinus arrhythmia in conscious humans. An important role for arterial carotid baroreceptors. *Circulation.* 1997; **95**: 1813–21.

CASE 3

Speed: 25 mm/s   Limb: 10 mm/mV   Chest: 10 mm/mV

Clinical scenario

Female, aged 36 years.

Presenting complaint
Palpitations.

History of presenting complaint
Six-month history of 'missed beats' occurring at rest,
particularly when lying quietly in bed. Symptoms are
more troublesome after drinking coffee.

Past medical history
Nil.

Examination
Pulse: 72 bpm, regular with occasional premature beat.
Blood pressure: 118/76.
JVP: not elevated.
Heart sounds: normal.
Chest auscultation: unremarkable.
No peripheral oedema.

Investigations
FBC: Hb 13.8, WCC 5.7, platelets 240.
U&E: Na 141, K 4.3, urea 2.8, creatinine 68.
Thyroid function: Normal.

Questions

1 What does this ECG show?
2 What advice would you offer?
3 Is any drug treatment required?

ECG analysis

Rate	72 bpm
Rhythm	Sinus rhythm with an atrial ectopic beat
QRS axis	Normal (+27°)
P waves	Present
PR interval	Normal (120 ms)
QRS duration	Normal (70 ms)
T waves	Normal
QTc interval	Normal (416 ms)

Additional comments

The P wave associated with the atrial ectopic beat is visible just towards the end of the preceding T wave.

Answers

1 This ECG shows normal sinus rhythm with a single **atrial ectopic beat** (the seventh beat along the rhythm strip).

2 The caffeine in coffee and in some cola drinks can be a trigger for atrial ectopic beats, and the patient should be advised to switch to decaffeinated alternatives. Other cardiac stimulants (such as alcohol and nicotine) can also act as triggers and should be moderated or avoided as appropriate.

3 Drug treatment is seldom required unless the atrial ectopic beats are particularly troublesome.

Commentary

● Atrial ectopic beats are also known as premature atrial complexes (PACs) or atrial extrasystoles. Atrial ectopic beats occur *earlier* than expected (in contrast with escape beats, which occur *later* than expected).

● Atrial ectopic beats can arise from any part of the atria, and the shape of the P wave depends upon where in the atria the ectopic has arisen from. In this patient's ECG, the P wave of the atrial ectopic beat has a shape very similar to the P wave of a normal sinus beat, suggesting an ectopic focus near to the sinoatrial node. In contrast, atrial ectopic beats that arise from low down in the atria, near the atrioventricular node, will have P waves that are inverted in the inferior leads but upright in lead aVR. This is because the wave of depolarization will predominantly move upwards in the atria, rather than downwards from the sinoatrial node. The P wave may also appear very close to, or overlapping with, the QRS complex, as a focus of depolarization near the atrioventricular node will reach the ventricles more quickly than one that has to travel from the sinoatrial node.

● Avoidance of triggers such as caffeine, alcohol and nicotine is often sufficient to reduce the frequency of atrial ectopic beats. They are generally benign, and so drug treatment is not usually needed unless the associated palpitations are very frequent and troublesome. If treatment is required, beta blockers can be effective in suppressing atrial ectopic activity.

Further reading
Making Sense of the ECG: Ectopic beats, p 61.

CASE 4

Clinical scenario

Female, aged 73 years.

Presenting complaint

Asymptomatic.

History of presenting complaint

Patient had recently moved house. She attended her new family doctor for a routine health check which included an ECG. Automated print-out reported 'Abnormal ECG'.

Past medical history

Mild hypertension.

Diet-controlled diabetes mellitus.

Osteoarthritis and bilateral hip replacements.

Examination

Pulse: 66 bpm, regular.

Blood pressure: 152/98.

JVP: not elevated.

Heart sounds: normal.

Chest auscultation: unremarkable.

No peripheral oedema.

Investigations

FBC: Hb 12.4, WCC 6.7, platelets 296.

U&E: Na 134, K 3.8, urea 5.1, creatinine 99.

Chest X-ray: normal heart size, clear lung fields.

Echocardiogram: Trivial mitral regurgitation into a non-dilated left atrium. Normal left ventricular function.

Questions

1 What does this ECG show?
2 What is the mechanism of this?
3 What are the likely causes?
4 What are the key issues in managing this patient?

ECG analysis

Rate	66 bpm
Rhythm	Sinus rhythm
QRS axis	Normal (+15°)
P waves	Normal
PR interval	Prolonged (240 ms)
QRS duration	Normal (100 ms)
T waves	Normal
QTc interval	Normal (420 ms)

Answers

1 The PR interval (which is measured from the start of the P wave to the start of the QRS complex) is greater than 200 ms, so conduction through the atrioventricular node is delayed; this delay is constant for each cardiac cycle. This is **first-degree atrioventricular block** ('first-degree heart block').

2 First-degree atrioventricular block is caused by delayed conduction of the atrial impulse to the ventricles through the atrioventricular node.

3 First-degree atrioventricular block can be a feature of ischaemic heart disease, hypokalaemia, acute rheumatic myocarditis, Lyme disease and drugs such as digoxin, beta blockers, some calcium channel blockers and quinidine. It can also be a normal physiological finding, particularly in young people with high vagal tone (e.g. during sleep).

4 First-degree atrioventricular block does not cause symptoms in its own right and does not usually require any specific intervention.

Commentary

● First-degree atrioventricular block is asymptomatic and no action is indicated. It rarely progresses to second or third-degree atrioventricular block. It should raise the possibility of one of the diagnoses listed above which may require treatment.

● First-degree atrioventricular block is not an indication for pacing.

Further reading

Making Sense of the ECG: First-degree atrioventricular block, p 118.

CASE 5

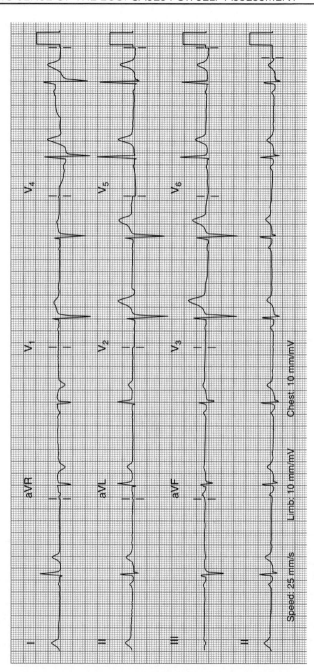

Speed: 25 mm/s   Limb: 10 mm/mV   Chest: 10 mm/mV

Clinical scenario

Male, aged 66 years.

Presenting complaint

Fatigue.

History of presenting complaint

The patient was diagnosed with hypertension six weeks ago and was commenced on treatment. Since that time he has felt tired and has noticed a reduction in his exercise capacity.

Past medical history

Hypertension, treated with atenolol 50 mg once daily.

Examination

Pulse: 42 bpm, regular.
Blood pressure: 156/94.
JVP: not elevated.
Heart sounds: normal.
Chest auscultation: unremarkable.
No peripheral oedema.

Investigations

FBC: Hb 13.8, WCC 7.6, platelets 313.
U&E: Na 138, K 4.2, urea 5.2, creatinine 98.

Questions

1 What rhythm is seen on this ECG?
2 What investigations would be appropriate?
3 What treatment is needed?
4 Is a pacemaker required?

ECG analysis

Rate	42 bpm
Rhythm	Sinus bradycardia
QRS axis	Normal (+1°)
P waves	Normal
PR interval	Normal (195 ms)
QRS duration	Normal (100 ms)
T waves	Normal
QTc interval	Normal (368 ms)

Answers

1 Sinus bradycardia, with a heart rate of 42 bpm.

2 In addition to the FBC and U&E listed, it would be appropriate to do thyroid function tests (to exclude hypothyroidism). An echocardiogram would determine whether left ventricular dysfunction is contributing to the patient's fatigue.

3 A reduction in the dose of the beta blocker, and possibly its complete withdrawal. Any reductions in beta blocker dose must be undertaken gradually to reduce the risk of 'rebound' tachycardia or hypertension.

4 A pacemaker is unlikely to be necessary – the clinical history makes it likely that the fatigue and bradycardia resulted from the recent introduction of a beta blocker, so the patient's fatigue should resolve on withdrawal of this.

Commentary

● Sinus bradycardia can be a normal finding in athletic individuals and also in most people during sleep.

● Always looks for correctable causes such as drug treatment (particularly beta blockers, digoxin or rate-limiting calcium channel blockers, such as verapamil). Do not forget about beta blocking eye drops, which can have systemic effects. Other causes include hypothyroidism, hypothermia, myocardial ischaemia and infarction, raised intracranial pressure (look for the combination of falling pulse and rising blood pressure), uraemia, obstructive jaundice and electrolyte abnormalities.

● Beta blockers are not recommended as first-line drugs for the management of hypertension, unless other indications exist, and so it would be appropriate to replace the beta blocker with an alternative drug in this case. A suitable choice for a hypertensive patient over the age of 55 years would be a calcium channel blocker or a thiazide diuretic.

● Permanent pacing is a treatment for symptomatic bradycardia, but it is essential to make sure that other correctable causes are identified and treated first – in this case, withdrawal of any negatively chronotropic drugs (those that slow the heart). Sometimes temporary transvenous pacing is required to support the patient, if he/she is severely symptomatic from their bradycardia, while any correctable causes are identified and treated.

Further reading

Making Sense of the ECG: Sinus bradycardia, p 31; Indications for temporary pacing, p 223; Indications for permanent pacing, p 225.

National Institute for Health and Clinical Excellence. *Management of hypertension in adults in primary care – updated guidance.* Clinical guideline 34. London: NICE, 2006. Available at www.nice.org.uk/guidance/CG34

CASE 6

Speed: 25 mm/s   Limb: 10 mm/mV   Chest: 10 mm/mV

Clinical scenario

Female, aged 79 years.

History of presenting complaint
Palpitations and breathlessness.

History of presenting complaint
The patient had been well until three days ago. She
noticed her heart beating faster when walking. She had
also started to struggle when doing housework.

Past medical history
Ischaemic heart disease for 10 years.
When she recently moved house and changed doctor,
her usual beta blocker was omitted in error from the
repeat prescription.

Examination
Pulse: 132 bpm, irregularly irregular.
Blood pressure: 120/70 approximately.

JVP: not seen (obese).
Heart sounds: normal.
Chest auscultation: fine basal crackles.
No peripheral oedema.

Investigations
FBC: Hb 11.7, WCC 5.6, platelets 310.
U&E: Na 141, K 4.3, urea 6.7, creatinine 124.
Thyroid function: normal.
Troponin I: negative.
Chest X-ray: mild cardiomegaly.
Echocardiogram: mild mitral regurgitation into non-
dilated left atrium. Left ventricular function mildly
impaired (ejection fraction 43 per cent).

Questions

1 What does this ECG show?
2 What is the mechanism of this?
3 What are the likely causes?
4 What are the key issues in managing this patient?

ECG analysis

Rate	136 bpm
Rhythm	Atrial fibrillation
QRS axis	Normal ($-4°$)
P waves	Absent
PR interval	N/A
QRS duration	Prolonged (140 ms)
T waves	Inverted (leads V_1–V_4)
QTc interval	Mildly prolonged (474 ms)

Additional comments

There is a right bundle branch block, which accounts for the T wave inversion.

Answers

1 The irregularly irregular rhythm with no discernible P waves means that this is **atrial fibrillation** (with a fast ventricular response). There is also right bundle branch block.

2 Atrial fibrillation results from rapid and chaotic atrial activity, with between 350 and 600 depolarizations per minute The atrioventricular node blocks some impulses and conducts others. The result is an irregularly irregular ventricular rhythm, the hallmark of atrial fibrillation.

3 There are many possible causes of atrial fibrillation. These include ischaemic heart disease, hypertension, valvular heart disease, hyperthyroidism, cardiomyopathy, sick sinus syndrome, thoracic surgery, acute and chronic alcohol misuse and constrictive pericarditis. Atrial fibrillation can also be idiopathic ('lone atrial fibrillation').

4 Patients with atrial fibrillation require a careful assessment to identify (and treat) the underlying cause. This includes a thorough history and examination, echocardiography, ambulatory ECG monitoring and blood tests (including thyroid function). Where required, ventricular rate control can be achieved with beta blockers, rate-limiting calcium channel blockers, digoxin or amiodarone. Risk stratify the patient with regard to thromboembolic risk and treat with warfarin or aspirin as appropriate. Decide whether attempting to restore (and maintain) sinus rhythm would be appropriate, or whether to accept atrial fibrillation and pursue a rate control strategy. Rhythm and rate control strategies are broadly equivalent with regard to mortality and quality of life.

Commentary

● Atrial fibrillation is common (the commonest sustained arrhythmia) and its prevalence increases with age.

● Atrial fibrillation may be:

- *Paroxysmal* – occurring intermittently and reverting spontaneously to sinus rhythm.
- *Persistent* – no period of sinus rhythm but no attempt at cardioversion to sinus rhythm has been made.
- *Permanent* – either atrial fibrillation is refractory and has resisted attempts or a decision has been made not to attempt to restore sinus rhythm.

● Atrial fibrillation may be asymptomatic, but can be accompanied by awareness of an irregular heartbeat, dyspnoea, fatigue, dizziness and syncope.

● In mitral stenosis, absolute risk of thromboembolism is 5–10 per cent per year untreated.

● In non-valvular atrial fibrillation, the absolute risk of stroke is 4 per cent per year untreated. The relative risk varies according to co-morbidity (with previous stroke/TIA 2.5× per decade; with diabetes 1.7× per decade; with hypertension 1.6× per decade; with increasing age 1.4× per decade).

● The annual thromboembolic risk can be reduced with warfarin: anticoagulated versus not anticoagulated = 1.4 per cent versus 4.5 per cent annual risk (68 per cent relative risk reduction overall).

Further reading

Making Sense of the ECG: Atrial fibrillation, p 42; Irregular cardiac rhythms, p 68.

National Institute for Health and Clinical Excellence. *The management of atrial fibrillation.* Clinical guideline 36. London: NICE, 2006. Available at www.nice.org.uk/guidance/CG36.

CASE 7

Speed: 25 mm/s   Limb: 10 mm/mV   Chest: 10 mm/mV

Clinical scenario

Male, aged 71 years.

Presenting complaint
Crushing central chest pain.

History of presenting complaint
Two-hour history of crushing central chest pain, which awoke the patient at 4.00 am. The pain radiates to the left arm and is associated with breathlessness, nausea and sweating.

Past medical history
Angina diagnosed 1 year ago.
Hypertension diagnosed 6 years ago.
Active cigarette smoker (48 pack-year smoking history).

Examination
Clammy, in pain.
Pulse: 85 bpm, regular.

Blood pressure: 148/82.
JVP: not elevated.
Heart sounds: normal.
Chest auscultation: unremarkable.
No peripheral oedema.

Investigations
FBC: Hb 13.8, WCC 10.2, platelets 349.
U&E: Na 138, K 4.2, urea 5.7, creatinine 98.
Troponin I: elevated at 23.4 (after 12 h).
Creatine kinase: elevated at 977 (after 12 h).
Chest X-ray: normal heart size, clear lung fields.
Echocardiogram: akinesia of inferior wall of left ventricle, overall ejection fraction 50 per cent.

Questions

1 What does this ECG show?
2 What other type of ECG recording should be performed? Why should this be done?
3 What treatment is indicated?
4 Should this ECG be repeated? When it should it be repeated and why?

ECG analysis

Rate	85 bpm
Rhythm	Sinus rhythm
QRS axis	Normal (+10°)
P waves	Present
PR interval	Normal (154 ms)
QRS duration	Normal (92 ms)
T waves	Lateral T inversion
QTc interval	Normal (428 ms)

Additional comments

There is ST segment elevation in the inferior leads (II, III, aVF) with reciprocal ST/T wave changes in the lateral leads (I, aVL, V_5–V_6).

Answers

1 This ECG shows an acute inferior ST segment elevation myocardial infarction (STEMI).

2 Another ECG should be performed immediately using right-sided chest leads (RV_1–RV_6) to look for evidence of right ventricular involvement in the inferior myocardial infarction.

3 Aspirin 300 mg orally (then 75 mg once daily), clopidogrel 300 mg orally (then 75 mg once daily for 1 month), glyceryl trinitrate sublingually, pain relief (diamorphine, plus an anti-emetic), oxygen. Prompt restoration of myocardial blood flow is required, either through primary percutaneous coronary intervention (PCI) or, if primary PCI is not available, thrombolysis.

4 Yes – if thrombolysis is used, the ECG must be repeated 90 min after the start of thrombolysis to determine whether coronary reperfusion has successfully been achieved. This is shown by resolution of the ST segment elevation by ≥50 per cent. In addition, whether primary PCI or thrombolysis is used, the ECG must be monitored throughout coronary reperfusion because of the risk of arrhythmias.

Commentary

● An urgent ECG is required in any patient presenting with cardiac-sounding chest pain. The presence of ST segment elevation signifies acute occlusion of a coronary artery and indicates a need for urgent restoration of coronary blood flow (reperfusion). This can be achieved with primary PCI or with thrombolysis. Time is of the essence – the longer reperfusion is delayed, the more myocardial necrosis will occur.

● The right ventricle is involved in 10–50 per cent of inferior ST segment elevation myocardial infarctions. It can be diagnosed by performing an ECG using right-sided chest leads (RV_1–RV_6) and looking for ST segment elevation in RV_4. Right ventricular infarction is important to recognize because it can have significant haemodynamic consequences. It may lead to signs of right heart failure (raised jugular venous pressure and peripheral oedema). If these patients develop hypotension, this may be because of failure of the right ventricle to pump sufficient blood to the left ventricle. Thus, despite the signs of right heart failure, it may be

necessary to give intravenous fluids to maintain left heart filling pressures. This is one situation in which haemodynamic monitoring with Swan–Ganz catheterization can prove helpful.

● A failure to achieve coronary reperfusion after thrombolysis may indicate the need to consider repeat thrombolysis or coronary angiography and 'rescue' PCI. If the ST segment elevation has not fallen by ≥50 per cent two hours after the start of thrombolysis, there is an 80–85 per cent probability that normal coronary blood flow has not been restored.

● The differential diagnosis of ST segment elevation includes acute myocardial infarction, left ventricular aneurysm, Prinzmetal's (vasospastic) angina, pericarditis, high take-off, left bundle branch block and Brugada syndrome.

Further reading

Making Sense of the ECG: Are the ST segments elevated? p 159; Why is right ventricular infarction important? p 167.
de Belder MA. Acute myocardial infarction: failed thrombolysis. *Heart* 2001; **81**: 104–12.

CASE 8

Clinical scenario

Male, aged 80 years.

Presenting complaint
Exertional chest pain, usually when walking uphill in cold and windy weather.

History of presenting complaint
Had been referred to hospital a few years ago with symptoms of exertional chest pain and diagnosed with angina.

Past medical history
Hypertension – well controlled.
Mild chronic airways disease.
Type 2 diabetes mellitus.
Is scheduled for prostatectomy – this ECG was recorded at preoperative assessment clinic.

Examination
Pulse: 84 bpm.
Blood pressure: 148/96.
JVP: not elevated.
Heart sounds: normal.
Chest auscultation: unremarkable.
No peripheral oedema.

Investigations
FBC: Hb 12.7, WCC 6.4, platelets 400.
U&E: Na 142, K 3.9, urea 6.5, creatinine 144.
Chest X-ray: mild cardiomegaly, early pulmonary congestion.
Echocardiogram: mildly impaired left ventricular function (ejection fraction 42 per cent).

Questions

1 What does this ECG show?
2 What is the underlying mechanism?
3 What are the likely causes?
4 What are the key issues in managing this patient?

ECG analysis

Rate	84 bpm
Rhythm	Sinus rhythm
QRS axis	Left axis deviation (−51°)
P waves	Normal
PR interval	Normal (160 ms)
QRS duration	Prolonged (125 ms)
T waves	Inverted in leads I, aVL, V_6
QTc interval	Mildly prolonged (460 ms)

Answers

1 This ECG shows sinus rhythm with broadened and notched QRS complexes (QRS duration >120 ms), QS in lead V_1 and a broad notched R wave in V_6: this is **left bundle branch block** (LBBB).

2 Left bundle branch block results from a failure of conduction in the left bundle branch. The left ventricle must be activated *indirectly* via the right bundle branch, so the right ventricle is activated before the left ventricle. This lengthens the overall duration of ventricular depolarization

and therefore broadens the QRS complexes (greater than 120 ms) and also distorts the QRS complexes. Repolarization is also abnormal, and ST segment depression and T wave inversion are frequently seen. Left bundle branch block may also be intermittent – especially in acute myocardial ischaemia. It may also occur with tachycardia (although rate-related bundle branch block more commonly causes right bundle branch block).

3 The causes of LBBB include ischaemic heart disease, cardiomyopathy, left ventricular hypertrophy (secondary to hypertension or aortic stenosis), fibrosis of the conduction system, myocarditis and rheumatic fever.

4 The presence of left bundle branch block is almost invariably pathological. Investigations are appropriate in the clinical context of chest pain, breathlessness and palpitations and also when LBBB is an incidental finding preoperatively. Investigations include echocardiography for cardiomyopathy and stress testing to identify myocardial ischaemia – dobutamine stress echo or nuclear myocardial perfusion imaging is appropriate, but avoid treadmill testing as LBBB distorts the ST segment.

Commentary

● Left bundle branch block is commonly seen in the elderly. In the absence of symptoms or when perioperative risk assessment is not warranted, no investigations are necessary.

Further reading

Making Sense of the ECG: Left bundle branch block, p 147; Causes of LBBB, p 152.

CASE 9

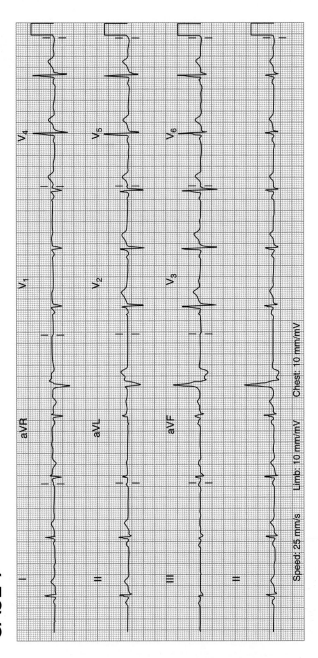

Speed: 25 mm/s   Limb: 10 mm/mV   Chest: 10 mm/mV

Clinical scenario

Male, aged 61 years.

Presenting complaint
Palpitations.

History of presenting complaint
Six-month history of intermittent palpitations, feeling like 'missed beats', particularly at rest. Otherwise asymptomatic. No chest pain, breathlessness, pre-syncope or syncope. No prolonged episodes of palpitation.

Past medical history
Nil.

Examination
Pulse: 60 bpm, occasional irregularity.
Blood pressure: 132/80.
JVP: not elevated.
Heart sounds: normal.
Chest auscultation: unremarkable.
No peripheral oedema.

Investigations
FBC: Hb 14.7, WCC 6.3, platelets 365.
U&E: Na 141, K 4.5, urea 4.8, creatinine 89.
Thyroid function: normal.
Chest X-ray: normal heart size, clear lung fields.

Questions

1 What rhythm is seen on this ECG?
2 What investigations might be appropriate?
3 What treatment options are available?

ECG analysis

Rate	60 bpm
Rhythm	Sinus rhythm with a single ventricular ectopic beat
QRS axis	Normal (+6°)
P waves	Present
PR interval	Normal (140 ms)
QRS duration	Normal (80 ms)
T waves	Normal
QTc interval	Normal (380 ms)

Answers

1 This ECG shows sinus rhythm with a single **ventricular ectopic beat** (VEB).

2 Ventricular ectopic beats are usually benign, but some patients may be at risk of dangerous ventricular arrhythmias. Assessment should include a full history and examination, and needs to be particularly thorough in those with structural heart disease or risk factors for sudden cardiac death (e.g. family history). Investigations may need to include a check of serum electrolytes, 12-lead ECG, echocardiography, ambulatory ECG monitoring (to quantify the frequency of VEBs and to screen for ventricular tachycardia) and exercise treadmill testing.

3 Identify and address any underlying causes (e.g. high caffeine intake, electrolyte abnormalities, myocardial ischaemia, cardiomyopathy). Benign VEBs may require just reassurance, although beta blockers may help if symptoms are troublesome. Patients at risk of dangerous arrhythmias may require catheter ablation or an implantable cardioverter defibrillator.

Commentary

● Ventricular ectopic beats, also known as ventricular premature complexes (VPCs) or ventricular extrasystoles, are a common finding and are often asymptomatic. They can, however, cause troublesome palpitations and sometimes herald a risk of dangerous arrhythmias. Patients with VEBs therefore require appropriate clinical assessment.

● VEBs cause broad QRS complexes and occur earlier than the next normal beat would have occurred. VEBs may be followed by inverted P waves if the atria are activated by retrograde conduction. If retrograde conduction does not occur, there will usually be a full compensatory pause before the next normal beat because the sinoatrial node will not be 'reset'.

● Two consecutive VEBs are termed a couplet; three or more are termed non-sustained ventricular tachycardia (lasting <30 s). VEBs with the same morphology are unifocal (arising from the same focus); those arising from multiple foci are termed multifocal.

● Causes of VEBs include structural heart disease (myocardial ischaemia/infarction, cardiomyopathy, valvular disease), electrolyte abnormalities, direct stimulation of the myocardium (e.g. pacing wires), some drugs (e.g. digoxin), caffeine, alcohol and sepsis.

● If VEBs are infrequent, and if heart disease and documented VT are absent, the prognosis is generally good.

● Beta blockers can be useful in those with troublesome symptoms but otherwise benign VEBs, although reassurance alone may suffice in this patient group. Where feasible, catheter ablation can be considered where symptoms are troublesome or there is a risk of malignant arrhythmias. An implantable cardioverter defibrillator is also an option to provide protection from dangerous arrhythmias.

Further reading

Making Sense of the ECG: Ventricular tachycardia, p 53; Ectopic beats, p 61.

Ng GA. Treating patients with ventricular ectopic beats. *Heart* 2006; **92**: 1707–12.

CASE 10

Speed: 25 mm/s   Limb: 10 mm/mV   Chest: 10 mm/mV

Clinical scenario

Female, aged 18 years.

Presenting complaint
Palpitations.

History of presenting complaint
Direct questioning reveals that the patient is aware of an episodic fast heart beat, particularly at times of stress and anxiety. Recently started studying at a local college and has been finding the coursework stressful.

Past medical history
Nil of note.

Examination
Pulse: 120 bpm.
Blood pressure: 118/76.

JVP: not elevated.
Heart sounds: normal.
Chest auscultation: unremarkable.
No peripheral oedema.

Investigations
FBC: Hb 12.9, WCC 6.5, platelets 356.
U&E: Na 141, K 4.1, urea 3.8, creatinine 86.
Thyroid function: normal.
Chest X-ray: normal heart size, clear lung fields.
Echocardiogram: normal valves and normal left ventricular function (ejection fraction 67 per cent).

Questions

1 What does this ECG show?
2 What are the likely causes?
3 What are the key issues in managing this patient?

ECG analysis

Rate	120 bpm
Rhythm	Sinus tachycardia
QRS axis	Normal (+35°)
P waves	Normal
PR interval	Normal (136 ms)
QRS duration	Normal (98 ms)
T waves	Normal
QTc interval	Normal (440 ms)

Answers

1 There is a normally shaped P wave before every QRS complex. This is **sinus tachycardia** (sinus rhythm with a heart rate greater than 100 bpm).

2 Sinus tachycardia is usually a normal physiological response to physical or emotional stress. There are numerous potential causes, including pain, anaemia, fever, dehydration, heart failure, hypotension, pulmonary embolism, drugs, exercise and anxiety. Sinus tachycardia may also result from thyrotoxicosis or drugs (e.g. beta agonists). Rarely it can be the result of a primary sinoatrial node abnormality (inappropriate sinus tachycardia).

3 First, it is important to establish that a tachycardia is indeed sinus tachycardia, as atrial tachycardia and atrial flutter can both resemble sinus tachycardia if the ECG is not inspected carefully enough. Second, a careful assessment of the patient is required to establish the cause of the sinus tachycardia and whether or not it is haemodynamically 'appropriate' (compensating for low blood pressure such as fluid loss or anaemia) or 'inappropriate' (e.g. anxiety, thyrotoxicosis). Third, although beta blockers are effective at slowing inappropriate sinus tachycardia, using a beta blocker to slow appropriate sinus tachycardia can lead to disastrous decompensation.

Commentary

● Clinical examination is essential. Thyroid function tests should always be requested. Catecholamine levels may be abnormal (phaeochromocytoma) – check especially if there is a history of hypertension.

● 'Palpitations' can be documented using:
  ● 12-lead ECG – most useful if the patient complains of palpitations during the recording.
  ● 24-h (or longer) ambulatory ECG recording – if palpitations are infrequent, the patient will have nothing to record.
  ● Cardiomemo – this patient-activated device may be carried for several weeks until an episode of palpitations occurs.
  ● Implantable loop recorder (Reveal device) – this is particularly useful if palpitations are infrequent but a serious arrhythmia is still suspected. The device is implanted subcutaneously and records the ECG continuously, storing periods that show arrhythmias or coincide with symptoms.

● Symptoms sometimes give a clue as to the underlying rhythm disturbance:
  ● Heart 'jumping' or 'missing a beat' – ectopics (atrial or ventricular).
  ● Intermittent rapid erratic heartbeat – paroxysmal atrial fibrillation.
  ● Sustained rapid regular palpitations with sudden onset and termination – atrioventricular re-entry tachycardia or atrioventricular nodal re-entry tachycardia.

Further reading

Making Sense of the ECG: Sinus tachycardia, p 32; Ambulatory ECG recording, p 232.

Morillo CA, Kleinm GJ, Thakur RK *et al.* Mechanism of 'inappropriate' sinus tachycardia. Role of sympathovagal balance. *Circulation* 1994; **90**: 873–3.

CASE 11

Clinical scenario

Male, aged 66 years.

Presenting complaint
Progressive exertional breathlessness.

History of presenting complaint
Normally active, he had noticed a gradual fall in his exercise capacity over a 2-week period prior to presentation. The main limiting factor in his exercise was breathlessness. He had not experienced any orthopnoea or paroxysmal nocturnal dyspnoea, and did not have any peripheral oedema.

Past medical history
Mitral valve prolapse with moderate mitral regurgitation.

Examination
Pulse: 75 bpm, regular.
Blood pressure: 118/78.

JVP: not elevated.
Heart sounds: 3/6 pansystolic murmur at apex, radiating to axilla.
Chest auscultation: bilateral inspiratory crackles at both lung bases.
No peripheral oedema.

Investigations
FBC: Hb 13.9, WCC 8.1, platelets 233.
U&E: Na 137, K 4.2, urea 5.3, creatinine 88.
Thyroid function: normal.
Troponin I: negative.
Chest X-ray: mild cardiomegaly, early pulmonary congestion.
Echocardiogram: Anterior mitral valve leaflet prolapse with posteriorly directed jet of moderate mitral regurgitation into a moderately dilated left atrium. Left ventricular function mildly impaired (ejection fraction 47 per cent).

Questions

1 What rhythm does this ECG show?
2 What is the mechanism of this arrhythmia?
3 How can the atrial rhythm be demonstrated more clearly?
4 What are the key issues in managing this arrhythmia?

ECG analysis

Rate	75 bpm
Rhythm	Atrial flutter
QRS axis	Normal (+68°)
P waves	Absent – atrial flutter waves are present
PR interval	Not applicable
QRS duration	Normal (80 ms)
T waves	Normal
QTc interval	Normal (358 ms)

Additional comments

The 'saw-tooth' pattern of atrial flutter is clearly evident, particularly in the inferior leads (II, III and aVF) and in chest lead V_1. There is one QRS complex for every 4 flutter waves (note that one flutter wave is masked by each QRS complex), indicating 4:1 atrioventricular block.

Answers

1 Atrial flutter with 4:1 atrioventricular block.

2 Atrial flutter usually results from a macro re-entry circuit within the right atrium (although other variants are recognized). The atria typically depolarize 300 times/min, giving rise to 300 flutter waves/min. However, depending on the type of atrial flutter, flutter rates can vary between 240 bpm and 430 bpm.

3 Flutter waves are best seen in the inferior leads and in lead V_1. They can be difficult to see when the ventricular rate is higher (e.g. with 2:1 or 3:1 block) as the flutter waves are masked by the overlying QRS complexes. Temporary blocking of the atrioventricular node with carotid sinus massage or adenosine (except where contraindicated) can block the QRS complexes for a few seconds, revealing the atrial activity more clearly.

4 There are four key aspects to the treatment of atrial flutter:

• Ventricular rate control – the drugs used for ventricular rate control are the same as those for atrial fibrillation (beta blockers or rate-limiting calcium channel blockers (e.g. verapamil, diltiazem), and/or digoxin).

• There is a thromboembolic risk, and patients should be considered for aspirin or warfarin in the same way as in atrial fibrillation.

• Electrical cardioversion can be very effective in restoring sinus rhythm and, as a general rule, atrial flutter is easier to cardiovert than atrial fibrillation.

• Electrophysiological intervention with ablation of the atrial flutter re-entry circuit is an effective procedure with a success rate greater than 90 per cent.

Commentary

● Atrial flutter is a common arrhythmia. It can occur in association with underlying cardiac disease such as ischaemic heart disease, valvular heart disease and cardiomyopathies, as well as in pulmonary diseases such as pulmonary embolism and chronic obstructive pulmonary disease.

● Although the atria depolarize around 300 times/min in atrial flutter, the atrioventricular node (fortunately) cannot conduct impulses to the ventricles that quickly, so after conducting an impulse the node will remain refractory for the next one, two or even more impulses until it is ready to conduct again. In this example, the node is conducting every fourth flutter wave to the ventricles, giving rise to 4:1 atrioventricular block.

● The heart rate will vary according to the degree of atrioventricular block – ventricular rates often run at 150 bpm (2:1 block), 100 bpm (3:1 block) or 75 bpm (4:1 block). The block can be variable, with a varying heart rate and an irregular pulse.

● Atrial flutter with 2:1 block is particularly common. In cases of 2:1 block the ventricular rate is around 150 bpm. Always consider a diagnosis of atrial flutter whenever someone presents with a regular narrow complex tachycardia and a ventricular rate of 150 bpm.

● The differential diagnosis of atrial flutter includes:
   ● Atrial tachycardia – The atrial rate is usually lower and the atrial activity is marked by abnormally shaped P waves rather than flutter waves.
   ● Atrial fibrillation – Can be mistaken for atrial flutter with variable block. Atrial activity in atrial fibrillation is less well defined on the ECG than the saw-tooth pattern seen in atrial flutter.

Further reading

Making Sense of the ECG: Atrial flutter, p 39.
Waldo AL. Treatment of atrial flutter. *Heart* 2000; **84**: 227–32.

CASE 12

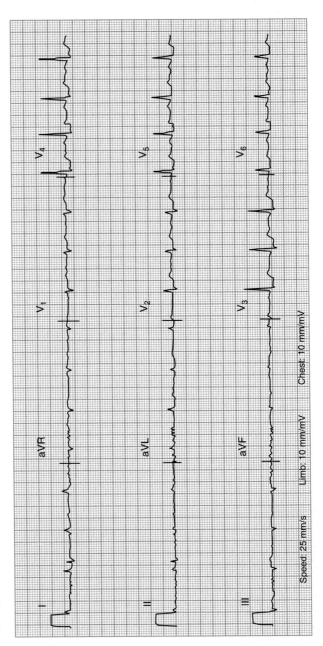

Speed: 25 mm/s   Limb: 10 mm/mV   Chest: 10 mm/mV

Clinical scenario

Male, aged 64 years.

Presenting complaint

Severe 'crushing' central chest pain.

History of presenting complaint

Chest pain on exertion for 3 months but put it down to indigestion. Tried over-the-counter antacids and pain eventually got better. However, he was then woken from sleep with severe chest pain. Started to have difficulty breathing.

Past medical history

Hypertension for 10 years.
Smoker of 30 cigarettes per day for 40 years.

Examination

Pulse: 90 bpm, regular.
Blood pressure: 156/104.

JVP: not elevated.
Heart sounds: normal.
Chest auscultation: unremarkable.
No peripheral oedema.

Investigations

FBC: Hb 15.5, WCC 6.9, platelets 198.
U&E: Na 139, K 5.1, urea 4.4, creatinine 96.
Thyroid function: normal.
Troponin I: normal (at 12 hours).
Chest X-ray: no cardiomegaly, mild pulmonary congestion.
Echocardiogram: normal valves. Mild concentric left ventricular hypertrophy. Left ventricular function mildly impaired (ejection fraction 46 per cent).

Questions

1 What does this ECG show?
2 What is the mechanism of this?
3 What are the key issues in managing this patient?

ECG analysis

Rate	90 bpm
Rhythm	Sinus rhythm
QRS axis	Normal (+14°)
P waves	Normal
PR interval	Normal (160 ms)
QRS duration	Normal (90 ms)
T waves	Normal
QTc interval	Normal (440 ms)

Additional comments

There is ST segment depression in leads V_2–V_6 and aVL.

Answers

1 The ECG shows sinus rhythm. There is ST segment depression in leads V_2–V_6 and aVL, indicating myocardial ischaemia in the territory of the left anterior descending coronary artery.

2 The mechanism of this ischaemia is likely to be a reduction in blood flow to the myocardium because of a degree of obstruction to flow down the left anterior descending coronary artery. In the view of the clinical presentation (acute coronary syndrome), it is likely that a previously stable coronary endothelial plaque has ruptured, exposing the lipid-rich core. Platelets adhere, change shape and secrete adenosine diphosphate (ADP) and other pro-aggregants; this may 'seal' and stabilize the plaque, but the lumen may be at least partially obstructed, reducing blood flow.

3 The patient should be admitted to a monitored area. Give pain relief with opiates with or without intravenous nitrates; beta blockers with or without calcium channel blockers; subcutaneous heparin; and anti-platelet treatment with aspirin and clopidogrel. Consider the use of an intravenous glycoprotein IIb/IIIa antagonist (e.g. tirofiban) to 'pacify' the culprit lesion. A troponin level should be checked to aid diagnosis and help formulate management. Arrange coronary angiography to define coronary anatomy. If a single 'culprit' lesion is identified, percutaneous coronary intervention (PCI) is effective. Complex lesions, including left main stem disease and bifurcation lesions, are increasingly treated with PCI, though multi-vessel disease is often treated with coronary bypass surgery.

Commentary

● Cardiac-sounding chest pain may be due to an acute coronary syndrome, classified on the basis of the ECG as:

● ST elevation acute coronary syndrome (STEACS): the ECG shows ST segment elevation and the primary aim of treatment is reopening of the coronary artery and reperfusion of the myocardium, via urgent primary PCI or thrombolysis depending on local availability.

● Non-ST elevation acute coronary syndrome (NSTEACS): the ECG may be normal, or may show ST segment depression or T wave inversion. The primary aim of treatment is urgent antiplatelet, antithrombotic and anti-ischaemic drug treatment, followed by coronary angiography as appropriate.

● The diagnosis of myocardial infarction is made later, once the troponin (I or T) results become available. The subgroup of patients with an elevated troponin level is classified as having had a myocardial infarction (either ST segment elevation myocardial infarction (STEMI) or non-ST segment elevation myocardial infarction

(NSTEMI)). Those whose troponin level remains normal retain the diagnostic label of acute coronary syndrome (troponin negative NSTEACS can also be referred to as unstable angina).

● The management of acute coronary syndromes has been driven by the results of randomized controlled clinical trials in which the treatment given reduced morbidity and mortality. What can be offered to patients depends on local facilities – transfer to a hospital with cardiac catheterization facilities may be necessary.

● As well as providing a useful diagnostic label, troponin results are helpful in allowing risk stratification – the degree of troponin elevation predicts a higher risk of future cardiovascular events.

Further reading

Making Sense of the ECG: Are the ST segments depressed? p 176; Acute coronary syndromes, p 189.

Fox KAA. Management of acute coronary syndromes: an update. *Heart* 2004; **90**: 698–706.

CASE 13

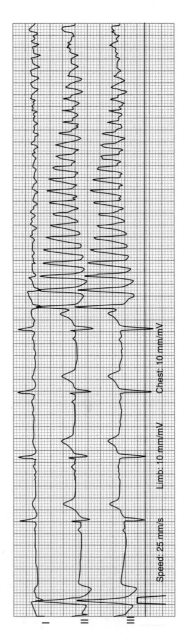

Speed: 25 mm/s   Limb: 10 mm/mV   Chest: 10 mm/mV

I

II

III

Clinical scenario

Male, aged 63 years.

Presenting complaint

Six-month history of worsening exertional chest pain.

History of presenting complaint

Strongly positive exercise treadmill test at low workloads for anterolateral ischaemia. Listed for urgent coronary angiography. This ECG was recorded during his coronary angiogram, which had revealed a severe left main stem coronary stenosis. The ECG shown above was recorded just after the first injection of contrast into the left coronary artery. The patient complained of chest pain, and then became unresponsive.

Past medical history

Angina.
Type 2 diabetes mellitus.
Hypertension.

Examination

Patient supine in cardiac catheter department, undergoing coronary angiography. Appears pale and clammy.
Blood pressure: 158/88, falling rapidly to become unrecordable while this ECG was recorded.
Patient became unresponsive during this ECG recording.

Investigations

FBC: Hb 14.1, WCC 7.6, platelets 304.
U&E: Na 139, K 4.4, urea 6.5, creatinine 84.
Glucose: 8.3 (known diabetes).

Questions

1 What does this ECG show?
2 What immediate action should be taken?
3 What medium-term action should be taken?

ECG analysis

Rate	52 bpm (during sinus rhythm), then unmeasurable
Rhythm	Sinus rhythm with ventricular ectopics, followed by ventricular tachycardia (VT) which rapidly degenerates into ventricular fibrillation (VF)
QRS axis	Left axis deviation (the axis moves increasingly leftward during the four sinus beats)
P waves	Present for the sinus beats, then absent during VT/VF
PR interval	Normal during sinus beats (160 ms)
QRS duration	Normal during sinus beats (110 ms)
T waves	Normal during sinus beats
QTc interval	Normal during sinus beats (392 ms)

Additional comments
The ventricular tachycardia is triggered by a ventricular ectopic beat occurring during the T wave of the fourth sinus beat (R on T ectopic).

Answers

1 The ECG shows a ventricular ectopic, followed by four normal sinus beats. Another ventricular ectopic beat then occurs during the T wave of the fourth sinus beat (R on T ectopic), triggering pulseless VT which then rapidly degenerates into VF.

2 The patient has sustained a cardiac arrest (pulseless VT/VF). As this was a witnessed and monitored arrest, a precordial thump can be given followed, if unsuccessful, by defibrillation with a DC shock. In this case, the patient did not respond to a precordial thump but sinus rhythm was restored following a single biphasic shock of 150 J. The patient should then be reassessed with regards to their airway, breathing and circulation.

3 Following successful resuscitation, the patient should be transferred to a coronary or intensive care unit for monitoring of airway and breathing (including pulse oximetry), vital signs (pulse, blood pressure (preferably via an arterial line) and temperature), peripheral perfusion, cardiac rhythm, neurological status (including Glasgow Coma Score) and urine output and fluid balance. In addition, check arterial blood gases, blood urea and electrolytes (including K^+, Mg^{2+} and Ca^{2+}), chest X-ray and blood glucose, 12-lead ECG and FBC.

In view of the critical nature of the patient's coronary disease, urgent revascularization should be arranged. Remember to speak to the patient's relatives as soon as possible after the cardiac arrest.

Commentary

● VF is characterized by its chaotic waveform with no discernible organized ventricular activity, in the context of a patient who is pulseless. A precordial thump is seldom successful in restoring sinus rhythm, but it is worth a single attempt at a precordial thump if the arrest was witnessed and monitored, and DC cardioversion is not immediately available. No time should be lost, however, in obtaining a defibrillator and administering a shock.

● Ventricular ectopic beats that fall on the T wave (R on T ventricular ectopics) occur during ventricular repolarization, which is a vulnerable time for ventricular arrhythmias. As the ventricles repolarize, they do so in a 'patchy' fashion, meaning that some areas of the myocardium repolarize more quickly than others. This leads to islands of refractory myocardium, surrounded by myocardium that has repolarized. A ventricular ectopic

arising at this time can establish a re-entry circuit around one of these refractory islands, causing VT which can then degenerate into VF.

● The ventricular ectopic beats and consequent pulseless VT/VF were, in this case, related to the patient's critical coronary disease. The left main stem is a critically important part of the coronary arteries and ischaemia or infarction arising from a left main stem stenosis will affect a large proportion of the left ventricle.

● Although arrhythmias account for 35 per cent of all complications during coronary angiography, they account for only 12 per cent of deaths, reflecting the careful monitoring of patients in the cardiac catheter department and the high level of expertise of staff in advanced life support.

Further reading

Making Sense of the ECG: Ventricular tachycardia, p 53; Ventricular fibrillation, p 57; Ectopic beats, p 61; Cardiopulmonary resuscitation, p 250.
Resuscitation Council (UK). Resuscitation guidelines. 2005. Available at: www.resus.org.uk.

CASE 14

V₁

II

V₅

Speed: 25 mm/s   Limb: 10 mm/mV   Chest: 10 mm/mV

Clinical scenario

Male, aged 66 years.

Presenting complaint
Sensation of 'missed heartbeats'.

History of presenting complaint
After retiring, and adopting a more sedentary lifestyle, the patient first became aware of something wrong when he was sitting quietly, reading the newspaper. He noticed that every now and then, his heart appeared to 'miss a beat'. Although he still enjoyed his normal weekend walking and badminton, he was anxious in case the missed beats were a sign of heart disease, as his mother had recently died of a 'massive heart attack'. He reported his concerns to his family doctor.

Past medical history
No significant medical history.

Examination
Pulse: 57 bpm, irregular (occasional 'missed beats').
Blood pressure: 144/94.
JVP: not elevated.
Heart sounds: normal.
Chest auscultation: unremarkable.
No peripheral oedema.

Investigations
FBC: Hb 14.3, WCC 7.5, platelets 278.
U&E: Na 139, K 5.0, urea 5.1, creatinine 96.
Chest X-ray: normal heart size, clear lung fields.
Echocardiogram: normal.

Questions

1 What does this ECG show?
2 What is the mechanism of this?
3 What are the likely causes?
4 What are the key issues in managing this patient?

ECG analysis

Rate	57 bpm
Rhythm	Sinus rhythm with second-degree atrioventricular block (Mobitz type I)
QRS axis	Unable to assess (rhythm strip)
P waves	Normal
PR interval	Variable – gradually lengthens before 'resetting' after a non-conducted P wave
QRS duration	Normal (110 ms)
T waves	Normal
QTc interval	Normal (400 ms)

Answers

1 The PR interval gradually increases after each successive P wave until one P wave is not conducted at all, resulting in a 'missed beat'. After this, conduction reverts to normal and the cycle starts over again. This is an example of second-degree atrioventricular block of the Mobitz type I (Wenckebach phenomenon) subtype.

2 The atrioventricular node 'fatigues' each time an impulse is conducted, until there is complete failure of conduction to the ventricles. After this period of 'rest', normal conduction is restored.

3 This manifestation of impaired conduction is benign. It may occur normally in sleep due to increased vagal tone and is a frequent normal finding on ambulatory ECG recordings in fit young people. It can also occur in disease of the conduction system.

4 The prognosis is good and no treatment is indicated unless symptomatic bradycardia occurs.

Commentary

● Mobitz type I or Wenckebach phenomenon is commonly reported in ambulatory ECG recordings during sleep. No action is required.

● 'Palpitations' can be difficult to document, especially if they are infrequent, of short duration or associated with sudden collapse. Options are:

● Prolonged (or repeated) Holter recording for 24 h, 48 h or 72 h duration – this will record every heart beat for a set period and will help determine whether the patient's perceived 'palpitation' is related to a cardiac problem. It is especially useful when symptoms occur on most days.

● If there are no events to record, the patient may be given a patient-activated Cardiomemo device – this can be carried for much longer periods (weeks if necessary) until the patient reports that a 'palpitation' has occurred.

● In a few patients, symptoms may still be suspected to be due to a cardiac arrhythmia but are not frequent enough for short ambulatory recordings to be practical. An implantable ECG loop recorder (Reveal device) may help. About the size and shape of a small computer 'memory stick', a loop recorder is implanted under local anaesthesia, just below the skin of the left chest wall. Although the device records continuously, the patient is taught how to electronically document when an event occurred so that the timing of the event can be checked against the cardiac rhythm at that time. The device can also automatically store rhythm strips when it detects a suspected rhythm disturbance.

Further reading

Making Sense of the ECG: Mobitz type I atrioventricular block, p 120; Indications for permanent pacing, p 225.

CASE 15

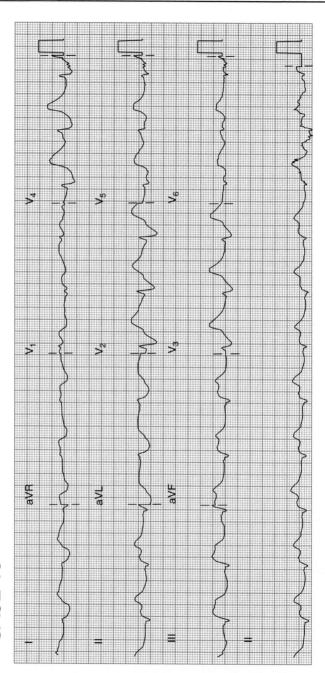

Clinical scenario

Female, aged 77 years.

Presenting complaint
Fatigue and feeling generally unwell.

History of presenting complaint
Known chronic renal impairment. One-week history of
diarrhoea and vomiting, with very poor fluid intake.
Presented with fatigue and feeling generally unwell.

Past medical history
Chronic renal impairment.

Examination
Patient appears dehydrated and unwell.
Pulse: 66 bpm, regular.
Blood pressure: 88/44.
JVP: low.
Heart sounds: normal.
Chest auscultation: unremarkable.
No peripheral oedema.
No urine output following urinary catheterization.

Investigations
FBC: Hb 10.8, WCC 22.1, platelets 211.
U&E: Na 130, K 8.2, urea 32.7, creatinine 642.

Questions

1 What does this ECG show?
2 What is the cause?

ECG analysis

Rate	66 bpm
Rhythm	Either sinus rhythm (with undetectable P waves) or junctional rhythm
QRS axis	Unable to assess in view of bizarre QRS complex morphology
P waves	Not visible
PR interval	Not applicable
QRS duration	Broad, bizarre complexes
T waves	Large, broad
QTc interval	Prolonged (>500 ms)

Answers

1 This ECG shows absent P waves and broad, bizarre QRS complexes. With increasing potassium levels, the P waves become smaller in size before disappearing altogether. Patients can also develop sinoatrial and atrioventricular block. The rhythm here may therefore be sinus rhythm with such small P waves that they are no longer evident, or a junctional rhythm (although junctional rhythms are usually slower).

2 The cause of these ECG appearances is severe hyperkalaemia – the patient's potassium level is markedly elevated at 8.2 mmol/L. This has developed as a result of acute-on-chronic renal failure, which is likely to have been precipitated by dehydration.

Commentary

● In general, hyperkalaemia causes a sequence of ECG changes at different potassium levels:

- early ECG changes include tall 'tented' T waves, shortening of the QT interval and ST segment depression
- at higher potassium levels, the QRS complexes become broad and there is lengthening of the PR interval (with flattening or even loss of the P wave)
- sinoatrial and atrioventricular block can develop
- at very high potassium levels, the QRS complexes become increasingly bizarre and merge with the T waves to resemble a sine wave
- arrhythmias (including ventricular fibrillation and asystole) can occur at any point.

● There is considerable variation in the ECG appearances between individuals with hyperkalaemia. Some patients will develop quite marked ECG abnormalities with fairly modest hyperkalaemia, while others can have minor ECG changes despite severe hyperkalaemia.

● Because of the risk of life-threatening arrhythmias, patients with hyperkalaemia need continuous ECG monitoring.

● If the diagnosis of hyperkalaemia is confirmed by an elevated plasma potassium level, assess the patient for symptoms and signs of an underlying cause (e.g. renal failure, as in this case). In particular, review their treatment chart for inappropriate potassium supplements and potassium-sparing diuretics.

● Hyperkalaemia needs urgent treatment if it is causing ECG abnormalities or the plasma potassium level is above 6.5 mmol/L.

Further reading

Making Sense of the ECG: Hyperkalaemia, p 187.
Webster A, Brady W, Morris F. Recognising signs of danger: ECG changes resulting from an abnormal serum potassium concentration. *Emerg Med J* 2002; **19**: 74–7.

CASE 16

Clinical scenario

Male, aged 26 years.

Presenting complaint
Asymptomatic.

History of presenting complaint
Incidental finding when attending for private insurance medical.

Past medical history
Nil of note.

Examination
Pulse: 66 bpm, regular.
Blood pressure: 126/84.
JVP: normal.
Heart sounds: normal.
Chest auscultation: unremarkable.
No peripheral oedema.

Investigations
FBC: Hb 16.2, WCC 6.4, platelets 332.
U&E: Na 141, K 4.9, urea 5.5, creatinine 90.
Chest X-ray: normal heart size, clear lung fields.
Echocardiogram: normal.

Questions

1 What does this ECG show?
2 What is the mechanism of this?
3 What are the possible causes?
4 What are the key issues in managing this patient?

ECG analysis

Rate	66 bpm
Rhythm	Sinus rhythm
QRS axis	Normal ($-24°$)
P waves	Normal
PR interval	Short (90 ms)
QRS duration	Lengthened (160 ms)
T waves	Normal
QTc interval	Normal (452 ms)

Additional comments

A delta wave is present (an initial slurred upstroke on the QRS complexes).

Answers

1 A P wave precedes every QRS complex so the rhythm is sinus rhythm. However, the PR interval is short, and there is slurring of the initial part of the QRS complex producing a delta wave, clearly visible in leads I, aVL and V_1–V_6. This is **Wolff–Parkinson–White (WPW) syndrome**.

2 Conduction from atria to ventricles is usually through a single connection involving the atrioventricular (AV) node and bundle of His. In WPW syndrome, a second accessory pathway (the bundle of Kent) coexists, and conducts an electrical signal from the atria to the ventricles at a faster rate than through the AV node, which means that the PR interval is shorter than normal. Also, the ventricles are activated by the accessory pathway before the impulse has (simultaneously) been transmitted through the AV node – known as ventricular pre-excitation. It causes the delta-shaped upstroke of the R wave. Eventually the impulse via the AV node catches up and fuses with the impulse depolarizing the ventricles via the accessory pathway, so that the remainder of ventricular depolarization occurs normally.

3 During fetal development, the atria and ventricles are separated electrically, with a single connection through the AV node and bundle of His. This protects the ventricles from rapid atrial activity, as the refractory period of the AV node places an upper limit on how rapidly atrial impulses can be transmitted to the ventricles. Incomplete separation leaves an accessory pathway, most often located in the left free wall or postero-septal wall, bypassing the AV node. Occasionally multiple pathways exist.

4 Patients may remain asymptomatic. Many patients with WPW syndrome experience episodes of atrioventricular re-entry tachycardia (AVRT), which can be treated pharmacologically or with ablation of the

accessory pathway. In the absence of palpitations, medical treatment and investigation is not necessary, but the individual should be advised to seek help immediately if palpitations occur.

Commentary

● Symptoms of AVRT are very variable. Patients complain of 'palpitations', usually of sudden onset and abrupt termination. The palpitations vary greatly in duration and severity, and may be accompanied by chest pain, dizziness or syncope.

● With anterograde conduction via the atrioventricular node and retrograde conduction via the accessory pathway, an orthodromic AVRT is said to occur. This is the commoner type of AVRT and during the tachycardia, the delta wave is lost. An AVRT taking the opposite route (down the accessory pathway and up the atrioventricular node) is said to be antidromic. This is rarer, and when it does occur, only delta waves are seen as the whole of the ventricular mass is activated via the accessory pathway.

● Some patients do not have any rhythm disturbance and the diagnosis of Wolff–Parkinson–White syndrome is made incidentally when an ECG is recorded for an unrelated problem. Patients should be encouraged to carry a copy of their 12-lead ECG in sinus rhythm – in the event of requiring surgery, it should be shown to the anaesthetist.

● Lown–Ganong–Levine syndrome (see Case 31) is another short PR syndrome but, unlike WPW syndrome, the accessory pathway does not activate ventricular muscle directly but instead connects the atria to the bundle of His. The wave of depolarization bypasses the slowly conducting AV node, causing a short PR interval *without* a delta wave. The risk of paroxysmal tachycardia is the same as in WPW syndrome.

Further reading

Making Sense of the ECG: AV re-entry tachycardias, p 46; Wolff–Parkinson–White syndrome, p 114.
Schilling RJ. Which patient should be referred to an electrophysiologist: supraventricular tachycardia. *Heart* 2002; **87**: 299–304.

CASE 17

Speed: 25 mm/s   Limb: 10 mm/mV   Chest: 10 mm/mV

Clinical scenario

Male, aged 37 years.

Presenting complaint
Severe central chest pain.

History of presenting complaint
Four-hour history of heavy central chest pain, radiating to the left arm and associated with breathlessness and sweating. Chest pain resolved after administration of opiates on arrival in hospital. This ECG was performed 24 h after presentation.

Past medical history
Hypertension diagnosed two years ago.
Ex-smoker (15 pack-year smoking history).

Examination
Pulse: 60 bpm, regular.
Blood pressure: 166/102.

JVP: not elevated.
Heart sounds: normal.
Chest auscultation: unremarkable.
No peripheral oedema.

Investigations
FBC: Hb 15.3, WCC 9.8, platelets 271.
U&E: Na 139, K 4.0, urea 5.8, creatinine 81.
Chest X-ray: normal heart size, clear lung fields.
Troponin I: elevated at 11.1 (after 12 h).
Creatine kinase: elevated at 532 (after 12 h).
Echocardiogram: hypokinesia of inferolateral walls of left ventricle, overall ejection fraction 50 per cent.

Questions

1 What abnormalities does this ECG show?
2 What is the diagnosis?
3 What treatment is indicated?

ECG analysis

Rate	60 bpm
Rhythm	Sinus rhythm
QRS axis	Normal (+73°)
P waves	Normal
PR interval	Normal (140 ms)
QRS duration	Normal (100 ms)
T waves	T wave inversion in leads II, III, aVF, V_5–V_6 and a biphasic T wave in lead V_4
QTc interval	Normal (420 ms)

Answers

1 This ECG shows inferolateral T wave inversion (leads II, III, aVF, V_5–V_6, with a biphasic T wave in lead V_4).

2 The ECG indicates an **inferolateral non-ST elevation acute coronary syndrome (NSTEACS)**. The elevated troponin I and creatine kinase levels confirm myocardial damage, and therefore a diagnosis of inferolateral non-ST segment elevation myocardial infarction (NSTEMI) can be made. In patients in whom the cardiac markers are not elevated 12 h after the onset of chest pain, myocardial infarction can be ruled out, and the diagnosis would be one of unstable angina.

3 The initial treatment of NSTEACS includes:

- aspirin
- clopidogrel
- heparin
- beta blocker
- nitrates
- statin
- oxygen and analgesia as appropriate.

High-risk patients may require a glycoprotein IIb/IIIa inhibitor. Patients may also require urgent coronary angiography with a view to coronary revascularization.

Commentary

● An urgent ECG is required in any patient presenting with cardiac-sounding chest pain. Acute coronary syndromes (ACS) can be divided into ST segment elevation ACS (STEACS) and non-ST segment elevation ACS (NSTEACS) on the basis of the ECG appearances. The ECG of a patient with NSTEACS may show ST segment depression, T wave inversion or may be normal.

● The differential diagnosis of T wave inversion includes:

● myocardial ischaemia
● myocardial infarction
● ventricular hypertrophy with 'strain'
● digoxin toxicity.

● T wave inversion is normal in leads aVR and V_1, and in some patients can be a variant of normal in leads V_2, V_3 and III. An inverted T wave is also normal in lead aVL if it follows a negative QRS complex.

● The location of ischaemic changes on an ECG is an indicator of the myocardial territory affected:

V_1-V_4	Anterior
I, aVL, V_5-V_6	Lateral
I, aVL, V_1-V_6	Anterolateral
V_1-V_3	Anteroseptal
II, III, aVF	Inferior
I, aVL, V_5-V_6, II, III, aVF	Inferolateral

● It is important to risk-stratify patients with ACS using a risk estimation tool, such as the TIMI Risk Score (www.timi.org). or the GRACE Registry Risk Score (www.outcomes-umassmed.org/grace), as this will help to guide the management strategy.

Further reading

Making Sense of the ECG: Are any of the T waves inverted? p 193.

Peters RJG, Mehta S, Yusuf S. Acute coronary syndromes without ST segment elevation. *BMJ* 2007; **334**: 1265–9.

CASE 18

Speed: 25 mm/s   Limb: 10 mm/mV   Chest: 10 mm/mV

Clinical scenario

Male, aged 44 years.

Presenting complaint

Awaiting minor surgery. Attended hospital for preoperative assessment.

History of presenting complaint

Asymptomatic: incidental finding.

Past medical history

Fit and well – keen tennis player.
No significant medical history.

Examination

Pulse: 66 bpm, regular.
Blood pressure: 134/90.
JVP: normal.
Heart sounds: normal.
Chest auscultation: unremarkable.
No peripheral oedema.

Investigations

FBC: Hb 16.1, WCC 5.7, platelets 320.
U&E: Na 140, K 4.7, urea 4.5, creatinine 94.
Chest X-ray: normal heart size, clear lung fields.
Echocardiogram: normal.

Questions

1 What does this ECG show?
2 What is the mechanism of this?
3 What are the likely causes?
4 What are the key issues in managing this patient?

ECG analysis

Rate	66 bpm
Rhythm	Sinus rhythm
QRS axis	Normal ($-11°$)
P waves	Normal
PR interval	Normal (180 ms)
QRS duration	Prolonged (140 ms)
T waves	Normal
QTc interval	Mildly prolonged (460 ms)

Additional comments

The QRS complexes have a right bundle branch block morphology.

Answers

1 The QRS complexes are broad (140 ms) and the QRS complex in lead V_1 has a rSR' ('M' shape) morphology. This is right bundle branch block (RBBB).

2 In RBBB the interventricular septum depolarizes normally from left to right. The electrical impulse then passes down the left bundle so the left ventricle depolarizes normally, but depolarization of the right ventricle is delayed because the depolarization has to occur via the left ventricle, travelling from myocyte to myocyte, rather than directly via the Purkinje fibres. This leads to a broad QRS complex with the characteristic rSR' morphology in lead V_1.

3 Right bundle branch block is a relatively common finding in normal hearts, but can be a marker of underlying disease including ischaemic heart disease, cardiomyopathy, atrial septal defect, Ebstein's anomaly, Fallot's tetralogy and pulmonary embolism (usually massive). It can also occur at fast heart rates in supraventricular tachycardia – this may lead to an incorrect diagnosis of ventricular tachycardia. Incomplete RBBB is found in 2–3 per cent of normal individuals and is usually of no clinical significance.

4 Right bundle branch block does not cause symptoms and does not require treatment. However, it is a prompt to look for an underlying cause. Investigations should be appropriate for the clinical presentation.

Commentary

● Right bundle branch block may be intermittent, occurring during episodes of tachycardia (when the heart rate exceeds the refractory period of the right bundle). Although both right and left bundle branch block can be 'rate related' in this way, the right bundle is more likely to be affected.

● An RBBB morphology is seen in Brugada syndrome, in association with persistent ST segment elevation in leads V_1–V_3. Brugada syndrome is an important diagnosis to make as it predisposes individuals to syncope and sudden death due to ventricular arrhythmias (see Case 68). It probably accounts for 50 per cent of sudden cardiac death with an apparently 'normal' heart. Although the ECG has an RBBB morphology in Brugada syndrome, this is not due to RBBB as such but rather is due to abnormal ventricular repolarization.

Further reading

Making Sense of the ECG: Right bundle branch block, p 148; Incomplete right bundle branch block, p 154; Brugada syndrome, p 176.

CASE 19

Speed: 25 mm/s   Limb: 10 mm/mV   Chest: 10 mm/mV

Clinical scenario

Male, aged 21 years.

Presenting complaint

Rapid regular palpitations.

History of presenting complaint

Normally fit and well with no prior history of palpitations. The patient presented with a 3 h history of rapid regular palpitation.

Past medical history

Wolff–Parkinson–White syndrome diagnosed at age 21 on a routine ECG at an insurance medical.

Examination

Pulse: 204 bpm, regular.
Blood pressure: 126/80.
JVP: normal.
Heart sounds: normal (tachycardic).
Chest auscultation: unremarkable.

Investigations

FBC: Hb 15.5, WCC 6.2, platelets 347.
U&E: Na 143, K 4.9, urea 4.6, creatinine 68.
Thyroid function tests: normal.
Chest X-ray: normal heart size, clear lung fields.

Questions

1 What does this ECG show?
2 What is the underlying pathophysiological mechanism?
3 What initial treatment would be appropriate?
4 What treatment might be appropriate in the longer term?

ECG analysis

Rate	204 bpm
Rhythm	Atrioventricular re-entry tachycardia (AVRT)
QRS axis	Unable to assess (single lead)
P waves	Inverted P waves after each QRS complex (distorting the ST segment/T wave)
PR interval	Not applicable
QRS duration	Normal (80 ms)
T waves	Distorted by inverted P waves
QTc interval	Normal (406 ms)

Answers

1 Atrioventricular re-entry tachycardia (AVRT).

2 A re-entry circuit involving an accessory pathway – in this case, the bundle of Kent in Wolff–Parkinson–White (WPW) syndrome. The re-entry circuit travels from atria to ventricles down through the atrioventricular node, as per normal, but then travels back up to the atria retrogradely via the accessory pathway. This is known as an orthodromic AVRT (in contrast to an antidromic AVRT, in which the re-entry circuit travels in the opposite direction, down the accessory pathway and back up the atrioventricular node).

3 Transiently blocking the atrioventricular node can terminate the AVRT. Methods to achieve this include:

- Valsalva manoeuvre
- carotid sinus massage
- intravenous adenosine
- intravenous verapamil.

4 The patient can be taught the Valsalva manoeuvre to try to terminate episodes. Treatment with maintenance anti-arrhythmic drugs (e.g. sotalol, verapamil, flecainide) can be used to try to prevent recurrent AVRT, but an electrophysiological study with a view to a radiofrequency ablation procedure is often preferable to long-term drug treatment in symptomatic patients.

Commentary

● Patients with WPW syndrome have an accessory pathway (the bundle of Kent) that provides an anatomical substrate for the development of AVRT. Not all patients with WPW syndrome will experience AVRT, however, and some can live out their full life without ever experiencing an episode of AVRT.

● Where WPW patients do get episodes of AVRT, this is usually orthodromic. Orthodromic AVRT is characterized by a narrow-complex tachycardia in which the delta wave is absent during the tachycardia (even though it is present during normal sinus rhythm) and the P waves are seen *after* the QRS complexes, and are inverted in the inferior leads. In the ECG presented here, inverted P waves can be seen at the junction of the ST segment and the T wave. The ECG appearances of antidromic AVRT are discussed in Case 59.

● AVRT is around 10 times less common than atrioventricular *nodal* re-entry tachycardia (AVNRT), which is caused by a micro re-entry circuit within the atrioventricular node. P waves are usually easier to discern in AVRT than in AVNRT, and the ECG in sinus rhythm in patients with a history of AVNRT is usually normal, but in those with a history of AVRT it may reveal a short PR interval or delta wave. The distinction between AVRT and AVNRT can be difficult, however, and may require electrophysiological studies.

Further reading

Making Sense of the ECG: atrioventricular re-entry tachycardias, p 47; Wolff–Parkinson–White syndrome, p 114.

Schilling RJ. Which patient should be referred to an electrophysiologist: supraventricular tachycardia. *Heart* 2002; **87**: 299–304.

CASE 20

Speed: 25 mm/s   Limb: 10 mm/mV   Chest: 10 mm/mV

Clinical scenario

Male, aged 75 years.

Presenting complaint

Syncope.

History of presenting complaint

Brought to emergency department feeling unwell after an episode of collapse with loss of consciousness. Reported several episodes of dizziness in past few months. Quickly back to normal within minutes but episodes tend to reoccur.

Past medical history

Osteoarthritis.

Examination

Pulse: 75 bpm, regular with occasional 'dropped beat'. Blood pressure: 156/96.

JVP: normal.
Heart sounds: normal.
Chest auscultation: unremarkable.
No peripheral oedema.

Investigations

FBC: Hb 13.9, WCC 8.1, platelets 233.
U&E: Na 137, K 4.2, urea 5.3, creatinine 88.
Thyroid function: normal.
Troponin I: negative.
Chest X-ray: normal.
Echocardiogram: normal.

Questions

1 What does this ECG show?
2 What are the likely causes?
3 What are the key issues in managing this patient?

ECG analysis

Rate	75 bpm
Rhythm	Sinus rhythm with intermittent sinoatrial node exit block
QRS axis	Unable to assess (rhythm strip)
P waves	Normal (when present)
PR interval	Normal (172 ms)
QRS duration	Normal (98 ms)
T waves	Normal
QTc interval	Normal (440 ms)

Answers

1 The underlying rhythm is normal sinus rhythm but then a P wave fails to appear; the next P wave appears after a pause of 2.4 s. The R-R interval is 0.8 s, so the P wave has arrived 'on schedule', three complete cycle lengths after the last P wave. This is **sinoatrial node exit block**, one of several types of sinus node dysfunction.

2 Sinoatrial node exit block may result from idiopathic fibrosis of the sinus node. Other causes include ischaemic heart disease, myocarditis, cardiomyopathy, cardiac surgery (especially atrial septal defect repair), drugs (such as beta blockers and rate-modifying calcium channel blockers) and digoxin toxicity, excessive vagal tone, and many ischaemic, inflammatory and infiltrative disorders.

3 Asymptomatic sinus node dysfunction does not require treatment. Any underlying causes should be addressed (e.g. drugs that can contribute to sinus node dysfunction should be withdrawn). Permanent pacing is appropriate for symptomatic patients (as in this example).

Commentary

● Sinoatrial node exit block should be distinguished from sinus arrest. In sinoatrial node exit block there is a pause with one or more absent P waves, and then the next P wave appears exactly where predicted – in other words, the sinoatrial node continues to 'keep time', but its impulses are not transmitted beyond the node to the atria. In sinus arrest, the node itself stops firing for a variable time period, so the next P wave occurs after a *variable* interval.

● Sinoatrial node exit block and sinus arrest can both be features of sinus node dysfunction (SND), formerly known as sick sinus syndrome. Other features of SND can include sinus bradycardia, brady-tachy syndrome and atrial fibrillation.

● Patients who drive a vehicle and who suffer from pre-syncope or syncope should receive appropriate advice about driving – very often, they will be barred from driving until the problem has been diagnosed and/or corrected as appropriate. Driving regulations vary between countries. In the UK, information on the medical aspects of fitness to drive can be found on the website of the Driver and Vehicle Licensing Agency (www.dvla.gov.uk).

Further reading
Making Sense of the ECG: Sinus arrest, p 35; Sinoatrial block, p 36.

CASE 21

Speed: 25 mm/s   Limb: 10 mm/mV   Chest: 10 mm/mV

Clinical scenario

Female, aged 78 years.

Presenting complaint

Exertional breathlessness and fatigue.

History of presenting complaint

One-year history of gradual onset exertional breathlessness and fatigue, with steady fall in exercise capacity.

Past medical history

Rheumatic fever aged 12 years.

Examination

Pulse: 84 bpm, regular.
Blood pressure: 118/70.

JVP: elevated by 2 cm.

Heart sounds: loud first heart sound (S_1) with an opening snap. Low-pitched 2/6 mid-diastolic murmur with pre-systolic accentuation heard at apex. Loud pulmonary component to second heart sound (P_2).

Chest auscultation: unremarkable.

Mild peripheral oedema.

Investigations

FBC: Hb 12.8, WCC 5.7, platelets 189.
U&E: Na 140, K 4.1, urea 3.7, creatinine 84.
Chest X-ray: large left atrium.

Questions

1 What does this ECG show?
2 What is the likely cause?
3 What would be the most helpful investigation?
4 What treatment is available?

ECG analysis

Rate	84 bpm
Rhythm	Sinus rhythm
QRS axis	Normal (+87°)
P waves	Broad, bifid
PR interval	Normal (150 ms)
QRS duration	Normal (100 ms)
T waves	Normal
QTc interval	Normal (450 ms)

Answers

1 The P waves are broad and bifid ('P mitrale').

2 In the clinical context, the most likely cause is left atrial enlargement secondary to rheumatic mitral stenosis. The clinical features are in keeping with severe mitral stenosis and associated pulmonary hypertension.

3 An echocardiogram would allow direct visualization of the mitral valve, measurement of left atrial size and an estimation of pulmonary artery pressure.

4 Correction of the mitral stenosis is indicated, using percutaneous balloon mitral valvuloplasty, surgical mitral valvotomy or mitral valve replacement.

Commentary

● P mitrale results from enlargement of the left atrium. The enlarged atrium takes longer to depolarize, and thus the P wave becomes broader. Although P mitrale does not require treatment in its own right, its presence should alert you to look for left atrial enlargement. This often results from mitral valve disease, but can also result from left ventricular hypertrophy (the elevated filling pressures of the 'stiff' left ventricle causes gradual enlargement of the left atrium).

● Decisions about which operative intervention to use in mitral stenosis depend primarily on the morphology of the mitral valve and its associated structures. Clear imaging of the valve is therefore essential, and most patients will require a transoesophageal echocardiogram to examine the valve in detail.

● Patients with severe mitral stenosis often develop atrial fibrillation. The consequent loss of P waves means that the ECG evidence of left atrial enlargement is lost.

Further reading

Making Sense of the ECG: Are any P waves too wide? p 109.
Prendergast BD, Shaw TRD, Iung B *et al.* Contemporary criteria for the selection of patients for percutaneous balloon mitral valvuloplasty. *Heart* 2002; **87**: 401–4.

CASE 22

Speed: 25 mm/s   Limb: 10 mm/mV   Chest: 10 mm/mV

Clinical scenario

Male, aged 56 years.

Presenting complaint

Episodes of irregular heart beat; occasionally feeling faint.

History of presenting complaint

For several weeks the patient had been afraid to leave his house due to frequent periods of feeling dizzy. Collapsed on two occasions, waking to find himself on the floor. Back to normal in minutes. Eventually sought advice of a doctor when he collapsed in the toilet and hit his head on the door.

Past medical history

Angina.
Hypertension.

Examination

Pulse: 66 bpm, regular with frequent 'dropped' beats.
Blood pressure: 156/86.
JVP: not elevated.
Heart sounds: normal.
Chest auscultation: unremarkable.
No peripheral oedema.

Investigations

FBC: Hb 12.2, WCC 8.4, platelets 342.
U&E: Na 137, K 4.2, urea 5.3, creatinine 88.
Thyroid function: normal.
Troponin I: negative.
Chest X-ray: normal heart size, clear lung fields.
Echocardiogram: structurally normal valves. Left ventricular function mildly impaired (ejection fraction 44 per cent).

Questions

1 What does this ECG show?
2 What is the mechanism of this?
3 What are the likely causes?
4 What are the key issues in managing this patient?

ECG analysis

Rate	66 bpm
Rhythm	Sinus rhythm with second-degree (Mobitz type II) atrioventricular block
QRS axis	Normal (+68°)
P waves	Normal
PR interval	140 ms (when P wave is followed by a QRS complex)
QRS duration	Normal (100 ms)
T waves	Normal
QTc interval	Normal (420 ms)

Answers

1 Most of the P waves are followed by a QRS complex with a normal and constant PR interval, but every third P wave is not followed by QRS complex. This is **second-degree atrioventricular block of the Mobitz type II type** – there is intermittent failure of conduction of atrial impulses *without a preceding lengthening of the PR interval*.

2 Second-degree atrioventricular block (Mobitz type II) results from intermittent failure of conduction of atrial impulses through the atrioventricular node. Mobitz type II block is usually due to infranodal block (i.e. below the atrioventricular node, whereas in Mobitz type I block, the block is confined to the atrioventricular node itself).

3 Causes of Mobitz type II atrioventricular block include idiopathic fibrosis of conducting tissue, acute myocardial infarction and drug-related conduction problems.

4 Mobitz type II atrioventricular block in acute infarction may progress unpredictably to complete heat block, so admission to a monitored area is mandatory:

- In acute **inferior** infarction, ischaemia is usually transient and a full recovery can be expected – resolution can be expected in hours or days but occasionally it may take 2–3 weeks. Temporary pacing is rarely needed.
- In acute **anterior** infarction, the combination of acute left ventricular dysfunction and a rhythm abnormality affects cardiac output markedly and mortality is increased considerably – temporary pacing may help increase cardiac output but does not alter outcome. Second-degree heart block due to chronic fibrosis is an indication for permanent pacing.

Commentary

- In Mobitz type II atrioventricular block:
  - The ratio of conducted to non-conducted atrial impulses varies but is commonly 2:1.
  - The atrial rate is normally regular (but occasionally it is not).
  - The risk of Stokes–Adams attacks (a sudden, transient episode of syncope in which the patient becomes pale and collapses due to a temporary pause in cardiac rhythm) is high. The episode may be confused with epilepsy – the patient may lie for several minutes motionless, pale and pulseless, but there is no incontinence or abnormal movements and recovery to normality is quick, often with flushing afterwards. A permanent pacemaker is curative.
  - There is a risk of slow ventricular rate and sudden death.

Further reading

Making Sense of the ECG: Mobitz type II AV block, p 121. Brignole M, Alboni P, Benditt DG *et al.* Guidelines on management (diagnosis and treatment) of syncope – update 2004. *Eur Heart J* 2004; **25**: 2054–72.

CASE 23

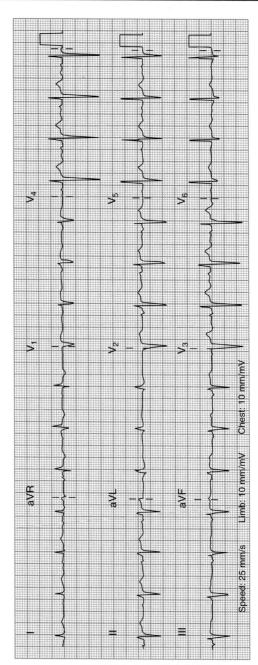

Speed: 25 mm/s   Limb: 10 mm/mV   Chest: 10 mm/mV

Clinical scenario

Female, aged 78 years.

Presenting complaint

Asymptomatic – routine ECG performed prior to orthopaedic surgery (right total hip replacement).

History of presenting complaint
No cardiac history as asymptomatic.

Past medical history
Osteoarthritis of the right hip.
No prior cardiac history.

Examination
Patient walks with a stick.
Comfortable at rest.
Pulse: 86 bpm, regular.
Blood pressure: 136/78.
JVP: not elevated.
Heart sounds: normal.
Chest auscultation: unremarkable.
No peripheral oedema.

Investigations
FBC: Hb 12.8, WCC 6.7, platelets 178.
U&E: Na 138, K 3.8, urea 5.7, creatinine 91.
Chest X-ray: normal heart size, clear lung fields.

Questions

1 What does this ECG show?
2 What can cause this?
3 Is any treatment necessary?

ECG analysis

Rate	86 bpm
Rhythm	Sinus rhythm
QRS axis	Left axis deviation (−51°)
P waves	Normal
PR interval	Normal (160 ms)
QRS duration	Normal (90 ms)
T waves	Normal
QTc interval	Normal (450 ms)

Answers

1 Left axis deviation (QRS axis −51°).

2 Left axis deviation can occur in normal individuals and as a result of:

- left anterior hemiblock
- inferior myocardial infarction
- Wolff–Parkinson–White syndrome
- chronic obstructive pulmonary disease.

3 Left axis deviation does not require treatment in its own right.

Commentary

● The normal QRS axis lies between −30° and +90° (although some cardiologists accept anything up to +120° as normal). Left axis deviation is conventionally diagnosed when the QRS axis lies more leftward (negative) than −30°.

● A quick way to assess QRS axis is to look at leads I and II:

• If the QRS complex is positive in leads I and II, then the axis is normal.

• If the QRS complex is positive in lead I and negative in lead II, then there is left axis deviation.

• If the QRS complex is negative in lead I and positive in lead II, then there is right axis deviation.

• Negative QRS complexes in both leads I and II most commonly indicate incorrect positioning of the limb electrodes and the ECG should be repeated.

● The left bundle branch divides into two sub-branches or fascicles – the left anterior fascicle and the left posterior fascicle. Block of the left anterior fascicle (left anterior hemiblock) can occur as a result of fibrosis of the conducting system (of any cause) or from myocardial infarction.

● On its own, left anterior hemiblock is not thought to carry any prognostic significance and no specific treatment is required. The presence of left axis deviation should not be a bar to orthopaedic surgery.

Further reading

Making Sense of the ECG: The axis, p 80; Is there left axis deviation? p 92.

CASE 24

Speed: 25 mm/s   Limb: 10 mm/mV   Chest: 10 mm/mV

Clinical scenario

Female, aged 80 years.

Presenting complaint

Nausea and vomiting.

History of presenting complaint

Patient has had atrial fibrillation for several years – not previously problematic. A week ago, felt generally unwell with mild fever and cough productive of green sputum. Family doctor prescribed antibiotics for a presumed respiratory tract infection. Although her symptoms were resolving, she stopped eating and drinking as she felt nauseous.

Past medical history

Rheumatic fever as child. Mixed mitral valve disease but symptoms not severe enough to warrant valve replacement surgery. Under regular follow-up with cardiologist.

Examination

Pulse: 72 bpm, irregularly irregular.
Blood pressure: 130/80.
JVP: not elevated.
Heart sounds: loud first heard sound; mid-diastolic rumble and pan-systolic murmur.
Chest auscultation: unremarkable.
Trace of ankle oedema.

Investigations

FBC: Hb 13.9, WCC 8.1, platelets 233.
U&E: Na 132, K 3.1, urea 8.9, creatinine 286.
Thyroid function: normal.
Troponin I: negative.
Chest X-ray: mild cardiomegaly.
Echocardiogram: thickened mitral leaflets with restricted movement; moderate mitral regurgitation into a moderately dilated left atrium. Left ventricular function mildly impaired (ejection fraction 43 per cent).

Questions

1 What does this ECG show?
2 Is this a sign of drug toxicity?
3 What mechanisms are involved?

ECG analysis

Rate	72 bpm
Rhythm	Atrial fibrillation
QRS axis	Normal (+47°)
P waves	Absent
PR interval	N/A
QRS duration	Normal (110 ms)
T waves	Inverted in most leads
QTc interval	Normal (440 ms)

Additional comments

There is downsloping 'reverse tick' ST segment depression in the inferior and anterolateral leads.

Answers

1 The rhythm is irregularly irregular with no discernible P waves (atrial fibrillation). The QRS complexes are normal but the ST segments are downward-sloping with a 'reverse tick' morphology: this is typical (although not diagnostic) of **digitalis (digoxin) effect**.

2 It is important to distinguish between the effects of digoxin on the ECG at normal therapeutic levels, and the effects of digoxin toxicity. ST segment depression is a normal finding in patients on digoxin, as is a reduction in T wave size and shortening of the QT interval. At toxic levels of digoxin, T wave inversion can occur, as can virtually any arrhythmia (but classically paroxysmal atrial tachycardia with atrioventricular block).

3 The effects of digoxin on the ECG are complex. It has a direct action by inducing electrical and mechanical effects by inhibiting sodium ion (and secondarily potassium ion) transport across myocardial and pacemaker cells, and an indirect effect by increasing vagal tone.

4 The most common ECG findings of digoxin toxicity are: heart block, bradycardia, junctional tachycardia and atrial fibrillation. Risk of digoxin toxicity increases with renal impairment, concomitant prescribing with verapamil or amiodarone, dehydration and hypokalaemia. The half-life of digoxin in normal renal function is 36–48 h, so in toxicity simply stopping the drug and supportive measures may be enough. It may be as long as 5 days in renal impairment. Digoxin is not removed by dialysis — if toxicity causes arrhythmias or malignant hyperkalaemia due to paralysed cell membrane-bound ATPase-dependent Na/K pumps), antibody fragments that bind with digoxin (Digibind) provide a specific antidote.

Commentary

● Causes of ST segment depression include drugs (digoxin, quinidine), myocardial ischaemia, acute posterior myocardial infarction, reciprocal changes in acute ST segment elevation myocardial infarction, and left ventricular hypertrophy with 'strain'.

● Always be careful to distinguish between ECG features seen with normal digoxin levels and those indicative of digoxin toxicity. Digoxin levels can be measured and guide clinical decision making.

● Symptoms of digoxin toxicity are non-specific: blurred vision, impaired colour perception (yellow or green vision was first reported by William Withering in 1785), confusion, anorexia, nausea, vomiting and diarrhoea.

● The risk of digoxin toxicity depends on the dose of digoxin, physical size of the patient, renal function and potassium level. Levels do not need to be routinely monitored but they are helpful if toxicity is suspected:

● <1.5 mcg/mL and normal K^+: toxicity unlikely
● 1.5–3.0 mcg/mL: toxicity possible
● >3.0 mcg/mL: toxicity likely

● Caution – always interpret digoxin levels in the light of clinical and chemical data.

Further reading

Making Sense of the ECG: Atrial fibrillation, p 42; Are the ST segments depressed? p 176; Digoxin and the ECG, p 180.

CASE 25

Clinical scenario

Female, aged 72 years.

Presenting complaint

Sudden onset breathlessness and pleuritic chest pain.

History of presenting complaint

Patient underwent left total knee replacement two days ago. Developed sudden onset breathlessness and right-sided pleuritic chest pain.

Past medical history

Left knee osteoarthritis.

Examination

Patient breathless at rest. In discomfort.

Pulse: 128 bpm, regular.

Blood pressure: 116/84.

JVP: elevated by 3 cm.

Heart sounds: gallop rhythm.

Chest auscultation: pleural rub heard in right mid-zone.

No peripheral oedema.

Investigations

FBC: Hb 11.8, WCC 11.1, platelets 323.

U&E: Na 141, K 4.3, urea 5.4, creatinine 95.

Chest X-ray: normal heart size, clear lung fields.

Questions

1 What does the ECG show?
2 What is the likely cause of this ECG appearance?
3 What investigations would be appropriate?
4 What are the treatment options?

ECG analysis

Rate	128 bpm
Rhythm	Sinus tachycardia
QRS axis	Normal (+16°)
P waves	Normal
PR interval	Normal (160 ms)
QRS duration	Normal (84 ms)
T waves	Inverted in leads III, aVF, V_1–V_4
QTc interval	Mildly prolonged (467 ms)

Additional comments
There is an $S_1Q_3T_3$ pattern and anterior T wave inversion.

Answers

1 This ECG shows:
  - sinus tachycardia
  - an S wave in lead I, and a Q wave and an inverted T wave in lead III ($S_1Q_3T_3$)
  - anterior T wave inversion.

2 Acute pulmonary embolism.

3 Appropriate investigations for suspected acute pulmonary embolism include:
  - arterial blood gases
  - chest X-ray (usually normal initially)
  - imaging studies: nuclear scintigraphy lung ventilation–perfusion (V/Q) scan; computed tomography (CT) pulmonary angiography.

4 The treatment of pulmonary embolism includes anticoagulation with heparin/warfarin, although thrombolysis may need to be considered in patients who have massive pulmonary embolism and/or are haemodynamically unstable. Oxygen therapy should be administered.

Commentary

● Sinus tachycardia is the commonest ECG abnormality found in pulmonary embolism.

● ECG indicators of right heart strain (pressure and/or volume overload) include the $S_1Q_3T_3$ pattern, also referred to as the McGinn–White sign (after Sylvester McGinn and Paul White, who first described the pattern in 1935). However, although the $S_1Q_3T_3$ pattern is often described as an indicator of pulmonary embolism, it is relatively insensitive and non-specific – it is only evident in around half of patients, and can occur in any condition that causes acute right heart strain (e.g. bronchospasm, pneumothorax).

● In those patients already suspected of having a pulmonary embolism, the presence of anterior T wave inversion has a sensitivity and specificity of >80 per cent for diagnosing massive pulmonary embolism.

● Other ECG abnormalities seen in pulmonary embolism can include incomplete right bundle branch block, P pulmonale (right atrial enlargement), non-specific ST segment changes and atrial fibrillation/flutter.

● A normal ECG does not exclude a diagnosis of pulmonary embolism.

Further reading

Making Sense of the ECG: Sinus tachycardia, p 32; $S_1Q_3T_3$ pattern, p 129.

Ferrari E, Imbert A, Chevalier T, *et al.* The ECG in pulmonary embolism. Predictive value of negative T waves in precordial leads – 80 case reports. *Chest* 1997; **111**: 537–43.

McGinn S, White PD. Acute cor pulmonale resulting from pulmonary embolism. Its clinical recognition. *JAMA* 1935; **104**: 1473–80.

CASE 26

Speed: 25 mm/s   Limb: 10 mm/mV   Chest: 10 mm/mV

Clinical scenario

Female, aged 69 years.

Presenting complaint
Breathless, especially going up stairs.

History of presenting complaint
Was fairly well until 3 months ago when a new family
doctor changed her medication.

Past medical history
Rheumatic fever.
Mitral regurgitation.

Examination
Pulse: 54 bpm, irregularly irregular.
Blood pressure: 110/70.
JVP: elevated by 2 cm.

Heart sounds: loud first sound, mitral regurgitation
easily heard.
Chest auscultation: unremarkable.
Mild pitting ankle oedema.

Investigations
FBC: Hb 12.6, WCC 5.9, platelets 345.
U&E: Na 133, K 4.1, urea 6.7, creatinine 168.
Thyroid function: normal.
Chest X-ray: mild cardiomegaly, early pulmonary
congestion.
Echocardiogram: thickened mitral leaflets, moderate
mitral regurgitation into a moderately dilated left
atrium. Left ventricular function mildly impaired
(ejection fraction 45 per cent).

Questions

1 What does this ECG show?
2 What is the mechanism of this?
3 What are the likely causes?

ECG analysis

Rate	54 bpm
Rhythm	Atrial fibrillation with a slow ventricular response
QRS axis	Normal (+31°)
P waves	Absent
PR interval	N/A
QRS duration	Normal (80 ms)
T waves	Normal
QTc interval	Normal (402 ms)

Answers

1 This ECG shows an irregularly irregular rhythm with absent P waves and a slow ventricular rate: this is **atrial fibrillation with a slow ventricular response**.

2 Atrial fibrillation with a slow ventricular response is usually due to an inappropriately high dose of an anti-arrhythmic agent (such as a beta blocker, rate-limiting calcium channel blocker or digoxin), although sometimes atrial fibrillation itself can occur with a relatively slow ventricular rate.

3 Many patients with atrial fibrillation are stable for years on their rate-controlling medication regimen but their ventricular rate control may be affected by:

- intercurrent illness – may cause an increased heart rate, e.g. respiratory infection
- drug compliance – failure to take as prescribed may cause inappropriately high or low drug levels
- changing renal function with age – affects the levels of drugs that are renally excreted
- gastrointestinal symptoms – may make absorption unpredictable
- initiation of other medication – some may increase digoxin levels (amiodarone, diltiazem, verapamil, spironolactone); some may reduce levels (antacids, sulphasalazine, metoclopramide, domperidone)

In this case, the cause of the 'slow' atrial fibrillation was a change in digoxin dose from 125 mcg to 250 mcg daily, despite the impaired renal function.

Commentary

● Always ensure that the rhythm has been diagnosed correctly before giving treatment – an inaccurate diagnosis means incorrect treatment that may cause symptoms to get worse.

● 'Slow' atrial fibrillation may not be easy to diagnose as the ECG baseline does not always show fibrillation waves and QRS complexes may look remarkably regular.

● Digoxin is renally excreted and has a half-life of 36 h. It has a narrow therapeutic 'window' and so caution must be taken in making dose adjustments in patients with renal impairment.

● The signs of digoxin toxicity include:
  ● cardiovascular – bradycardia (<60 bpm), atrioventricular conduction block, supraventricular tachycardia, ventricular extrasystoles
  ● central nervous system – dizziness, confusion, nightmares, hallucinations
  ● visual – yellowing of vision, halo effect
  ● gastrointestinal – anorexia, nausea, vomiting, diarrhoea, abdominal pain.

Further reading

Making Sense of the ECG: Atrial fibrillation, p 42.

CASE 27

Speed: 25 mm/s   Limb: 10 mm/mV   Chest: 10 mm/mV

Clinical scenario

Male, aged 57 years.

Presenting complaint

Sudden collapse.

History of presenting complaint

Patient admitted for investigation of right calf tenderness and swelling. Collapsed suddenly in the X-ray department immediately after he arrived for a leg ultrasound Doppler. This rhythm strip was recorded on arrival of the cardiac arrest team.

Past medical history

Patient had been resting at home following a right leg injury 3 weeks earlier.

Examination

Unresponsive – Glasgow Coma Scale score 3/15.
Pulse: unrecordable – pulses not palpable.
Blood pressure: unrecordable.
JVP: neck veins distended.
No respiratory movements.
Right calf red and swollen.

Investigations

FBC: Hb 14.1, WCC 10.6, platelets 306.
U&E: Na 137, K 4.1, urea 6.7, creatinine 112.
Chest X-ray: normal heart size, clear lung fields.

Questions

1 What does this ECG rhythm strip show?
2 What is the clinical diagnosis, and the likely underlying cause?
3 What action should be taken?

ECG analysis

Rate	108 bpm
Rhythm	Sinus tachycardia
QRS axis	Unable to assess (single lead)
P waves	Normal
PR interval	Normal (195 ms)
QRS duration	Normal (80 ms)
T waves	Normal
QTc interval	Mildly prolonged (456 ms)

Answers

1 This ECG rhythm strips shows sinus tachycardia, 108 bpm.

2 The patient has collapsed and is unconscious (Glasgow Coma Scale score 3/15) with no detectable cardiac output. This is therefore a cardiac arrest with **pulseless electrical activity (PEA)**, sometimes also called electromechanical dissociation (EMD). The likely cause in this clinical context is **massive pulmonary embolism,** secondary to a deep vein thrombosis of the right leg.

3 Standard basic and advanced life support algorithms should be followed. Pulseless electrical activity is a non-shockable rhythm and it is particularly important to look for an underlying treatable cause.

Commentary

- Pulseless electrical activity occurs when the heart is still working electrically but is failing to produce an output.
- It is important to remember that PEA can be seen in conjunction with *any* cardiac rhythm that would normally sustain a circulation. The diagnosis of PEA is therefore not an ECG diagnosis *per se* (the ECG can look entirely normal), but is based upon the clinical context of a patient with no cardiac output despite a heart that appears to be working electrically.
- Causes of PEA include:
  - hypoxia
  - hypovolaemia
  - hyperkalaemia, hypokalaemia, hypocalcaemia, acidaemia, and other metabolic disorders
  - hypothermia
  - tension pneumothorax
  - tamponade
  - toxic substances
  - thromboembolism (pulmonary embolus/coronary thrombosis).
- Pulseless electrical activity is managed according to the non-shockable rhythms (PEA and asystole) treatment algorithm of the Resuscitation Council (UK).

Further reading

Making Sense of the ECG: Cardiopulmonary resuscitation, p 250; Pulseless electrical activity, p 260.
Resuscitation Council (UK). Resuscitation guidelines. 2005. Available at: www.resus.org.uk

CASE 28

Speed: 25 mm/s   Limb: 10 mm/mV   Chest: 10 mm/mV

Clinical scenario

Female, aged 76 years.

Presenting complaint

Woken from sleep with severe chest pain.

History of presenting complaint

Had angina on exertion for over 4 years. Similar pain to usual angina but much worse. Never had pain at rest or at night before – felt like there was 'someone sitting on my chest'. The pain radiated to the left arm and was associated with breathlessness. She was afraid she might die.

Past medical history

Hypertension – well controlled on amlodipine and bendroflumethiazide.

Diabetes mellitus.

Hypercholesterolaemia.

Ex-smoker. Strong family history of coronary artery disease.

Examination

Pulse: 66 bpm, regular.
Blood pressure: 182/98.
JVP: not elevated.
Heart sounds: soft pansystolic murmur at apex (mitral regurgitation).
Chest auscultation: bilateral basal crackles.
No peripheral oedema.

Investigations

FBC: Hb 11.5, WCC 5.2, platelets 401.
U&E: Na 132, K 4.5, urea 7.0, creatinine 131.
Troponin I: elevated at 10.5 (after 12 h).
Chest X-ray: mild cardiomegaly, early pulmonary congestion.
Echocardiogram: mild mitral regurgitation. Left ventricular function mildly impaired (ejection fraction 47 per cent).

Questions

1 What does this ECG show?
2 What is the mechanism of this?
3 What are the likely causes?
4 What are the key issues in managing this patient?

ECG analysis

Rate	66 bpm
Rhythm	Sinus rhythm
QRS axis	+70°
P waves	Normal
PR interval	Normal (160 ms)
QRS duration	Normal (96 ms)
T waves	Merged with ST segment
QTc interval	Normal (420 ms)

Additional comments
There is ST segment elevation in the lateral leads (I, aVL, V_4–V_6).

Answers

1 There is ST segment elevation in limb leads I and aVL and chest leads V_4–V_6. This is an **acute lateral ST elevation myocardial infarction** (STEMI).

2 Acute occlusion of the diagonal branch of the left coronary artery.

3 A previously stable coronary endothelial plaque has ruptured, exposing the lipid-rich core. Platelets adhere, change shape and secrete adenosine diphosphate (ADP) and other pro-aggregants. These seal and stabilize the plaque but at the cost of narrowing of the coronary artery lumen. This is often totally, or almost totally, occluded.

4 Treatment is aimed at restoring coronary patency. This can be achieved by:

• Primary percutaneous coronary intervention (PCI) in the catheter laboratory

• Thrombolysis, using an intravenous thrombolytic to break down the thrombus and reopen the occluded coronary artery.

Immediate management also includes pain relief (morphine or diamorphine plus an anti-emetic) and antiplatelet therapy (aspirin with or without clopidogrel) should be given. The patient should be admitted to a monitored area to treat any complications (heart failure, potentially lethal arrhythmia). Secondary prevention (angiotensin-converting enzyme (ACE) inhibitor, beta blocker, statin and anti-smoking advice). Remember to provide primary prevention advice to family members.

Commentary

● An urgent ECG is required in any patient presenting with cardiac-sounding chest pain. The presence of ST segment elevation signifies acute occlusion of a coronary artery and indicates a need for urgent restoration of coronary blood flow (reperfusion). This can be achieved with primary PCI or with thrombolysis. Time is of the essence – the longer reperfusion is delayed, the more myocardial necrosis will occur.

● The management of acute coronary syndrome has been driven by the results of randomized controlled clinical trials showing reduction in mortality and morbidity using a combination of thrombolysis, anti-platelet drugs, early coronary angiography and coronary angioplasty (with or without a stent) or coronary bypass surgery. What can be offered to patients depends on local facilities – transfer to a hospital with cardiac catheterization facilities may be necessary. In some countries, all patients with acute coronary syndrome are admitted to a dedicated 'heart attack centre' where diagnostic coronary angiography and percutaneous intervention can be made available 24 h a day.

● A failure to achieve coronary reperfusion after thrombolysis may indicate the need to consider repeat thrombolysis or coronary angiography and 'rescue' PCI. If the ST segment elevation has not fallen by ⩾50 per cent within 90 minutes after the start of thrombolysis, there is an 80–85 per cent probability that normal coronary blood flow has not been restored.

● The differential diagnosis of ST segment elevation includes acute myocardial infarction, left ventricular aneurysm, Prinzmetal's (vasospastic) angina, pericarditis, high take-off, left bundle branch block and Brugada syndrome.

Further reading

Making Sense of the ECG: Are the ST segments elevated? p 159.

Task Force on the Management of Acute Myocardial Infarction of the European Society of Cardiology. Management of acute myocardial infarction in patients presenting with ST-segment elevation. *Eur Heart J* 2003; **24**: 28–66.

de Belder MA. Acute myocardial infarction: failed thrombolysis. *Heart* 2001; **81**: 104–12.

CASE 29

Speed: 25 mm/s   Limb: 10 mm/mV   Chest: 10 mm/mV

Clinical scenario

Female, aged 23 years.

Presenting complaint
Rapid regular palpitations.

History of presenting complaint
Two-year history of episodic rapid regular palpitations, normally lasting only a few minutes, with a sudden onset and termination. The current episode started suddenly 2 h prior to presentation.

Past medical history
Nil.

Examination
Pulse: 180 bpm, regular.
Blood pressure: 112/72.
JVP: normal.
Heart sounds: normal (tachycardic).
Chest auscultation: unremarkable.

Investigations
FBC: Hb 13.5, WCC 5.2, platelets 302.
U&E: Na 140, K 4.4, urea 4.5, creatinine 73.
Chest X-ray: normal heart size, clear lung fields.

Questions

1 What does this ECG show?
2 What is the underlying pathophysiological mechanism?
3 What initial treatment would be appropriate?
4 What treatment might be appropriate in the longer term?

ECG analysis

Rate	180 bpm
Rhythm	Atrioventricular nodal re-entry tachycardia
QRS axis	Normal (+22°)
P waves	Visible as a small negative deflection at the end of the QRS complex in the inferior leads
PR interval	Not applicable
QRS duration	Normal (60 ms)
T waves	Normal
QTc interval	Normal (450 ms)

Answers

1 Atrioventricular nodal re-entry tachycardia (AVNRT).
2 A re-entry circuit involving a dual atrioventricular nodal pathway – one of the atrioventricular nodal pathways conducts impulses quickly (the 'fast' pathway) but has a long refractory period, the other pathway conducts impulses more slowly (the 'slow' pathway) but has a shorter refractory period (see Commentary).

3 Transiently blocking the atrioventricular node can terminate the AVNRT. Methods to achieve this include:

- Valsalva manoeuvre
- carotid sinus massage
- intravenous adenosine
- intravenous verapamil.

4 The patient can be taught the Valsalva manoeuvre to try to terminate episodes. Recurrent AVNRT may require treatment with anti-arrhythmic drugs (e.g. sotalol, verapamil, flecainide) or an electrophysiological study with a view to a radiofrequency ablation procedure.

Commentary

● In patients with a dual atrioventricular nodal pathway, an impulse arriving at the atrioventricular node will normally split and travel down both pathways at the same time, but the impulse travelling via the fast pathway arrives at the bundle of His first and depolarizes the ventricles. By the time the impulse travelling down the slow pathway arrives at the bundle of His, the bundle is refractory and so this impulse goes no further.

● However, if a supraventricular ectopic beat happens to occur during the refractory period of the fast pathway, this ectopic will travel down the slow pathway and, by the time it reaches the end of the slow pathway, the fast pathway may have repolarized. If so, this impulse will then travel back *up* along the fast pathway, and then back down the slow pathway, ad infinitum. In the common form of AVNRT, this slow-fast re-entry circuit gives rise to the arrhythmia. Fast-slow and slow-slow re-entry circuits are also possible.

● In AVNRT, P waves are often hard or even impossible to discern. In around a quarter of cases, they are hidden within the QRS complexes. In another two-thirds of cases, they can be seen as a small negative deflection at the end of the QRS complexes in the inferior leads, and/or as a small positive deflection at the end of the QRS complex in lead V_1. In a small number of cases, the P wave can be found just before the QRS complex.

● AVNRT is around 10 times commoner than atrioventricular re-entry tachycardia (AVRT – the result of an atrioventricular accessory pathway as seen in Wolff–Parkinson–White syndrome). The ECG in sinus rhythm in AVNRT is usually normal, but in AVRT an ECG in sinus rhythm may reveal a short PR interval or delta wave, suggesting Wolff–Parkinson–White syndrome. The distinction between AVRT and AVNRT can be difficult, however, and may require electrophysiological studies.

Further reading

Making Sense of the ECG: Atrioventricular re-entry tachycardias, p 47.
Schilling RJ. Which patient should be referred to an electrophysiologist: supraventricular tachycardia. *Heart* 2002; **87**: 299–304.

CASE 30

Speed: 25 mm/s   Limb: 10 mm/mV   Chest: 10 mm/mV

Clinical scenario

Male, aged 84 years.

Presenting complaint
Increasing exertional breathlessness.

History of presenting complaint
Had been fairly well until developed chest infection.
Breathlessness has got progressively worse since.

Past medical history
Previous rheumatic fever.

Examination
Pulse: 42 bpm, irregular.
Blood pressure: 122/76.
JVP: normal.
Heart sounds: normal.
Chest auscultation: unremarkable.
No peripheral oedema.

Investigations
FBC: Hb 11.1, WCC 4.7, platelets 224.
U&E: Na 135, K 4.7, urea 5.8, creatinine 146.
Thyroid function: normal.
Troponin I: negative.
Echocardiogram: awaited.

Questions

1 What does this ECG show?
2 What is the mechanism of this?
3 What are the likely causes?
4 What are the key issues in managing this patient?

focus away from the sinoatrial node. Only some of the P waves are followed by QRS complexes, and the QRS rate is variable. This is **atrial tachycardia with variable atrioventricular block.**

2 Atrial tachycardia results from increased automaticity of a focus of depolarization in the atria. The variable atrioventricular block is due to depressed conduction through the atrioventricular node.

3 The presence of 'reverse tick' lateral ST segment depression suggests that the patient is taking digoxin, and indeed this arrhythmia proved to be the result of digoxin toxicity.

4 Temporary (and occasionally permanent) withdrawal of digoxin treatment. Supportive measures until digoxin levels have fallen to therapeutic levels or symptoms of nausea have ceased. An alternative anti-arrhythmic drug may be required.

ECG analysis

Rate	42 bpm
Rhythm	Atrial tachycardia with variable atrioventricular block
QRS axis	+80°
P waves	Present but abnormal morphology
PR interval	N/A
QRS duration	Normal (80 ms)
T waves	Abnormal
QTc interval	Normal (350 ms)

Additional comments

The P waves are abnormally shaped, indicating an atrial focus away from the sinoatrial node, and the P wave rate is 156 bpm (but most P waves are not conducted to the ventricles). There is also a partial RBBB pattern and lateral ST segment depression.

Answers

1 This ECG shows regular P waves at a rate of 156 bpm. The P waves have an abnormal morphology, indicating a

Commentary

● In atrial tachycardia, the ventricular rate depends upon the degree of atrioventricular block. With 1:1 conduction, the ventricular rate may be rapid.

● Atrial tachycardia may occur in tachy-brady syndrome, rheumatic and ischaemic heart disease, chronic airways disease and cardiomyopathy.

● Digoxin affects the heart in various ways:
  ● an inotropic effect through inhibition of the sodium/potassium/ATPase pump
  ● increased automaticity of Purkinje fibres
  ● slowing of conduction through the atrioventricular node due to increased vagal activity.

● With digoxin toxicity, increased automaticity results in an increased atrial rate and slowing of conduction induces atrioventricular block and subsequent slowing of the ventricular rate.

● Toxicity can occur with digoxin levels within the therapeutic range if there is severe hypokalaemia (often due to diuretic therapy) or renal impairment.

● Although paroxysmal atrial tachycardia with variable block is considered the 'hallmark' of digoxin toxicity, in clinical practice the arrhythmia is often sustained. In addition, digoxin can cause almost any cardiac arrhythmia.

Further reading

Making Sense of the ECG: Atrial tachycardia, p 37; Effects of digoxin on the ECG, p 180.

CASE 31

Speed: 25 mm/s   Limb: 10 mm/mV   Chest: 10 mm/mV

Clinical scenario

Male, aged 29 years.

Presenting complaint
Episodic palpitations.

History of presenting complaint
A 2-year history of rapid regular palpitations, occurring once a week on average and lasting for between 10 and 60 minutes. Prolonged episodes are associated with dizziness.

Past medical history
Nil.

Examination
Pulse: 66 bpm, regular with infrequent ectopics.
Blood pressure: 132/82.
JVP: not elevated.
Heart sounds: normal.
Chest auscultation: unremarkable.
No peripheral oedema.

Investigations
FBC: Hb 14.5, WCC 5.7, platelets 286.
U&E: Na 141, K 4.6, urea 4.1, creatinine 72.
Thyroid function: normal.
Chest X-ray: normal heart size, clear lung fields.

Questions

1 What does this ECG show?
2 What is the likely cause of the patient's palpitations?
3 What further investigations would be appropriate?

ECG analysis

Rate	66 bpm
Rhythm	Sinus rhythm with a single supraventricular ectopic beat
QRS axis	Normal (+0°)
P waves	Normal
PR interval	Short (100 ms)
QRS duration	Normal (76 ms)
T waves	Normal
QTc interval	Normal (450 ms)

Additional comments
The PR interval is short at 100 ms.

Answers

1 The ECG shows a short PR interval, measuring 100 ms (2.5 small squares). In the context of episodic palpitations, this is suggestive of a diagnosis of Lown–Ganong–Levine (LGL) syndrome. The diagnosis can be confirmed by demonstrating the occurrence of episodes of atrioventricular re-entry tachycardia.

2 The presence of an accessory pathway in LGL syndrome allows for an atrioventricular re-entry tachycardia.

3 The patient's ECG should be recorded during an episode of palpitation in order to make a diagnosis of atrioventricular re-entry tachycardia and thus to confirm LGL syndrome. Ambulatory ECG recording can be used. As the patient's symptoms are occurring once a week on average, a 7-day ECG event recorder or a Cardiomemo would be the most effective ways of trying to capture an event.

Commentary

● The diagnosis of LGL syndrome requires the presence of a short PR interval (<120 ms), a normal QRS complex duration and episodes of atrioventricular re-entry tachycardia.

● The presence of a short PR interval *in the absence of* any history of palpitations is not sufficient for a diagnosis of LGL syndrome, and may indicate a normal variant of accelerated conduction through the atrioventricular node rather than the presence of an accessory pathway.

● LGL syndrome has often been described as being due to an accessory pathway that connects the atria to the bundle of His. Although several such pathways have been identified, such as James fibres, no single anatomical substrate specific to LGL syndrome has been found. The anatomical basis of LGL syndrome has therefore been the subject of debate, with many questioning whether it is a specific entity in its own right or whether it is simply a clinical manifestation of a range of different atrioventricular conduction anomalies.

Further reading

Making Sense of the ECG: Lown–Ganong–Levine syndrome, p 117.

Lown B, Ganong WF, Levine SA. The syndrome of short P-R interval, normal QRS complex and paroxysmal rapid heart action. *Circulation* 1952; **5**: 693.

CASE 32

Speed: 25 mm/s   Limb: 10 mm/mV   Chest: 10 mm/mV

Clinical scenario

Male, aged 74 years.

Presenting complaint

Admitted to hospital with chest pain and breathlessness on exertion.

History of presenting complaint

Symptom-free until 3 months ago. Developed chest pain on exertion, especially if walking uphill, in cold weather or when wind blowing. Occasionally had chest pain at rest, requiring glyceryl trinitrate spray. Pain was gradually getting worse. Had one episode of chest pain that woke him the night before admission.

Past medical history

History of hypertension and hypercholesterolaemia. Acute myocardial infarction 3 years ago, treated with thrombolysis. Chronic bronchitis on home nebulizers.

Examination

Pulse: 120 bpm, regular with occasional ectopic beats. Blood pressure: 152/92.

JVP: not elevated.

Heart sounds: soft ejection systolic murmur in aortic area, radiating to neck.

Chest auscultation: unremarkable.

No peripheral oedema.

Investigations

FBC: Hb 12.9, WCC 6.5, platelets 342.

U&E: Na 136, K 4.7, urea 5.1, creatinine 132.

Troponin I: negative.

Chest X-ray: mild cardiomegaly, early pulmonary congestion.

Echocardiogram: mild aortic stenosis, with pressure drop of 20 mmHg across valve, mild mitral regurgitation into a non-dilated left atrium. Left ventricular function mildly impaired (ejection fraction 43 per cent) with anterior wall akinesia.

Questions

1 What does this ECG show?
2 What is the mechanism of this?
3 What are the likely causes?
4 What are the key issues in managing this patient?

ECG analysis

Rate	120 bpm
Rhythm	Sinus tachycardia with occasional atrial ectopic beats
QRS axis	+53°
P waves	Normal
PR interval	Normal (180 ms)
QRS duration	Normal (80 ms)
T waves	Normal
QTc interval	Normal (440 ms)

Additional comments

Anterior Q waves (leads V_1–V_3).

Answers

1 There are Q waves in the anterior chest leads V_1–V_3, indicative of a previous anterior myocardial infarction. Q waves are considered 'pathological' if they exceed two small squares in depth, or are greater than 25 per cent of the size of the following R wave, and/or are greater than 1 small square wide.

2 Previous acute occlusion of the left anterior descending coronary artery.

3 Rupture of coronary atheroma, platelet activation and thrombus formation. Thrombolysis may restore coronary patency by dissolving thrombus overlying a ruptured coronary plaque but does not affect the size of the underlying coronary plaque. With progression of atheromatous deposition despite secondary preventive measures, flow past the coronary plaque slowly declines until physical activity leads to an imbalance between myocardial demand and supply and consequently the onset of symptoms.

4 If symptomatic, investigate for myocardial ischaemia – conduct an exercise treadmill test, stress echocardiogram, stress cardiac magnetic resonance (MR) scan or nuclear myocardial perfusion scan. If myocardial ischaemia is evident, especially at low cardiac workload, arrange coronary angiography to define the coronary anatomy and to identify potential targets for revascularization by percutaneous coronary intervention (PCI) or bypass surgery. Secondary prevention (aspirin, clopidogrel, beta blocker, angiotensin-converting enzyme (ACE) inhibitor and statin) should be considered for all patients with a previous history of myocardial infarction.

Commentary

● This patient clearly has a history of coronary artery disease, in view of the previous myocardial infarction, and presents with a clinical history consistent with unstable angina (cardiac-sounding chest pain and negative troponin).

● A patient referred for 'routine' surgery may report a previous myocardial infarction or an ECG may show evidence of an 'old' (previously undiagnosed) myocardial infarction. The risk of an adverse perioperative event is increased with:

● known coronary disease, especially within three months of a myocardial infarction
● previously unidentified coronary disease
● valvular heart disease, especially aortic stenosis
● cardiac arrhythmia
● heart failure/cardiogenic shock
● co-morbidity

● coronary risk factors indicating high risk of coronary disease
● renal impairment
● abnormal liver function
● previous stroke or transient ischaemic attack (TIA)
● poor exercise tolerance.

● Several indices are available to assess perioperative risk (see Further reading).

Further reading

Making Sense of the ECG: The Q wave, p 127; Evolution of a Q wave myocardial infarction, p 161.

Detsky AS, Abrams HB, Forbath N *et al*. Cardiac assessment for patients undergoing non-cardiac surgery. A multifactorial clinical risk index. *Arch Intern Med* 1986; **146**: 2131–4.

Mangano DT, Goldman L. Preoperative assessment of patients with known or suspected coronary disease. *N Engl J Med* 1995; **333**: 1750–6.

CASE 33

Speed: 25 mm/s   Limb: 10 mm/mV   Chest: 10 mm/mV

Clinical scenario

Female, aged 86 years.

Presenting complaint
Dizziness and syncope, breathlessness.

History of presenting complaint
Four-day history of increasing breathlessness and dizziness, culminating in an episode of syncope in which the patient suddenly fell to the floor with little warning.

Past medical history
Myocardial infarction 2 months earlier.
Type 2 diabetes mellitus.

Examination
Pulse: 32 bpm, regular.
Blood pressure: 108/60.
JVP: elevated by 2 cm, intermittent cannon waves.
Heart sounds: variable intensity of second heart sound.
Chest auscultation: few bi-basal inspiratory crackles.
Mild peripheral oedema.

Investigations
FBC: Hb 12.1, WCC 6.3, platelets 206.
U&E: Na 136, K 4.2, urea 4.8, creatinine 81.
Thyroid function: normal.
Chest X-ray: cardiomegaly, pulmonary vascular congestion.

Questions

1 What does this ECG show?
2 What are the possible causes?
3 What treatment is required?

ECG analysis

Rate	Atrial – 90 bpm
	Ventricular – 32 bpm
Rhythm	Third-degree atrioventricular block (complete heart block')
QRS axis	Can't be measured (single lead)
P waves	Present
PR interval	Variable – no apparent connection between P waves and QRS complexes
QRS duration	Prolonged (140 ms)
T waves	Inverted in leads III, aVF, V$_1$–V$_4$
QTc interval	Prolonged (475 ms)

Answers

1 Third-degree atrioventricular block ('complete heart block').

2 Third-degree atrioventricular block can result from:
- ischaemic heart disease
- fibrosis and calcification of the conduction system (Lev's disease)
- drugs that block the atrioventricular node (e.g. beta blockers, calcium channel blockers, digoxin – especially in combination)
- Lyme disease
- acute rheumatic fever
- congenital complete heart block.

3 Third-degree atrioventricular block associated with symptoms requires pacing.

Commentary

● In third-degree atrioventricular block (complete heart block'), there is complete interruption of conduction between atria and ventricles, so that the two are working independently. The atrial (P wave) rate is faster than the ventricular (QRS complex) rate, and the P waves bear no relationship to the QRS complexes.

● QRS complexes usually arise as the result of a ventricular escape rhythm. The QRS complexes are usually broad due to a subsidiary pacemaker ('escape rhythm') arising in the left or right bundle branches. However, if the atrioventricular block occurs high up in the conduction system (at the level of the atrioventricular node) and a subsidiary pacemaker aries in the bundle of His, the QRS complexes may be narrow.

● Any atrial rhythm can coexist with third-degree heart block, and so the P waves may be abnormal or even absent.

● In the context of an acute **inferior** wall myocardial infarction, third-degree atrioventricular block requires

pacing if the patient is symptomatic or haemodynamically compromised. In acute **anterior** wall myocardial infarction, the development of third-degree atrioventricular block usually indicates an extensive infarct, and temporary pacing is indicated regardless of the patient's symptoms or haemodynamic state.

● Temporary pacing is usually necessary perioperatively in patients about to undergo surgery who are found to have third-degree atrioventricular block.

Further reading

Making Sense of the ECG: Third-degree atrioventricular block, p 123; Pacemakers and implantable cardioverter defibrillators, p 222.

Gammage MD. Temporary cardiac pacing. *Heart* 2000; **83**: 715–20.

Morgan JM. Basics of cardiac pacing: selection and mode choice. *Heart* 2006; **92**: 850–4.

CASE 34

Speed: 25 mm/s   Limb: 10 mm/mV   Chest: 10 mm/mV

Clinical scenario

Male, aged 69 years.

Presenting complaint

Feeling generally weak and lethargic. Also had frequent palpitations.

History of presenting complaint

Fit and well until about 3 months ago when diagnosed with hypertension and commenced on a thiazide diuretic.

Past medical history

Hypertension.

Examination

Pulse: 84 bpm, regular.
Blood pressure: 136/88.

JVP: normal.
Heart sounds: normal.
Chest auscultation: unremarkable.
No peripheral oedema.

Investigations

FBC: Hb 14.7, WCC 5.6, platelets 168.
U&E: Na 136, K 2.8, urea 4.6, creatinine 76.
Thyroid function: normal.
Chest X-ray: normal heart size, clear lung fields.
Echocardiogram: normal valves. Concentric left ventricular hypertrophy.

Questions

1 What does this ECG show?
2 What is the mechanism of this?
3 What are the likely causes?
4 What are the key issues in managing this patient?

ECG analysis

Rate	84 bpm
Rhythm	Sinus rhythm
QRS axis	Borderline left axis deviation (−30°)
P waves	Small but normal morphology
PR interval	Prolonged (400 ms)
QRS duration	Normal (80 ms)
T waves	Normal
QTc interval	Normal (390 ms)

Answers

1 This ECG shows first-degree atrioventricular block (long PR interval), small T waves and there are U waves evident. These findings are secondary to **hypokalaemia.** There is also left axis deviation.

2 Depolarization of myocardial cells is dependent on the movement of ions across the cell membrane, the most important being potassium. The resting transmembrane potential is determined largely by the ratio of the intracellular (140 mmol/L) potassium ion concentration to extracellular (3.5 to 5 mmol/L) potassium ion concentration, and the absolute level of extracellular potassium ion concentration is the most important factor affecting the cell membrane.

3 Thiazide diuretic therapy, vomiting and diarrhoea, excessive perspiration, rectal villous adenoma, intestinal fistula, Cushing's and Conn's syndromes, alkalosis, purgative and laxative misuse, renal tubular failure, hypomagnesaemia (usually evident when K^+ remains low after potassium supplementation). Rare causes include Bartter's syndrome (hereditary defect of muscular ion channels) and hypokalaemic periodic paralysis.

4 If hypokalaemia is suspected, assess the patient for symptoms (such as muscle weakness and cramps) and enquire about prescribed drugs (diuretics are a common cause). Mild hypokalaemia can be corrected with dietary or oral supplements. Severe hypokalaemia is a medical emergency and should be corrected with slow intravenous infusion of appropriately diluted potassium chloride via a central line – fast or concentrated infusions may predispose to ventricular tachycardia.

Commentary

● Mild hypokalaemia may occur without symptoms. Moderate hypokalaemia may cause muscle weakness, cramps and constipation. With more severe hypokalaemia, flaccid paralysis, hyporeflexia, respiratory depression and tetany may be seen.

● Hypokalaemia is much more common than hyperkalaemia and can produce the following ECG changes:

- ST segment depression
- decreased T wave amplitude
- increased U wave amplitude
- prolonged QT interval
- less commonly (and more subtly) prolonged QRS duration and increased P wave amplitude and duration.

● Resulting instability of cell membranes causes an increased risk of cardiac arrhythmia, especially atrial and ventricular ectopic beats, atrial and ventricular tachycardia, various heart blocks and ventricular fibrillation.

● Hypomagnesaemia is common with hypokalaemia; alone, it causes similar ECG abnormalities. Hypokalaemia is often difficult to correct until the magnesium level is normal.

● Caution – digoxin toxicity is more likely with hypokalaemia.

● It is important to measure serum potassium in all cases of suspected myocardial infarction. Although distinct changes may be observed, the ECG is not a reliable indicator of potassium level.

Further reading

Making Sense of the ECG: Hypokalaemia, p 191; Do the U waves appear too prominent? p 214.

CASE 35

Speed: 25 mm/s   Limb: 10 mm/mV   Chest: 10 mm/mV

Clinical scenario

Male, aged 48 years.

Presenting complaint
Asymptomatic – routine ECG performed during hypertension follow-up visit.

History of presenting complaint
Six-year history of hypertension, treated with an angiotensin-converting enzyme (ACE) inhibitor.

Past medical history
Six-year history of hypertension.

Examination
Patient comfortable at rest.
Pulse: 66 bpm, regular.

Blood pressure: 168/104.
JVP: not elevated.
Precordium: left parasternal heave.
Heart sounds: loud aortic component of second heart sound (A_2).
Chest auscultation: unremarkable.
No peripheral oedema.

Investigations
FBC: Hb 15.8, WCC 7.0, platelets 314.
U&E: Na 140, K 4.4, urea 6.2, creatinine 101.
Chest X-ray: normal heart size, clear lung fields.

Questions

1 What does the ECG show?
2 What investigation would help to confirm this?
3 What can cause these appearances? What is the likely cause here?
4 What are the treatment options?

ECG analysis

Rate	66 bpm
Rhythm	Sinus rhythm
QRS axis	Normal (+48°)
P waves	Normal
PR interval	Normal (167 ms)
QRS duration	Normal (96 ms)
T waves	Normal
QTc interval	Normal (420 ms)

Additional comments

In the chest leads there are deep S waves (up to 15 mm in lead V_2) and tall R waves (up to 39 mm) in lead V_4.

Answers

1 This ECG shows deep S waves (up to 15 mm in lead V_2) and tall R waves (up to 39 mm) in lead V_4 in the chest leads. These appearances are indicative of left ventricular hypertrophy. The diagnostic criteria in this case include:

• R wave in lead V_4 measuring 39 mm
• S wave in lead V_1 plus R wave in lead V_5 totalling 41 mm

• Tallest R wave and deepest S wave in chest leads totalling 54 mm.

2 An echocardiogram (or cardiac magnetic resonance scan) would allow direct visualization of the left ventricle, assessment of the extent of left ventricular hypertrophy, assessment of left ventricular systolic (and diastolic) function, and also assessment of the heart valves.

3 Left ventricular hypertrophy can result from:

• hypertension
• aortic stenosis
• coarctation of the aorta
• hypertrophic cardiomyopathy.

The clinical findings indicate that poorly controlled hypertension is the most likely cause of left ventricular hypertrophy in this case.

4 Where left ventricular hypertrophy is secondary to pressure overload of the left ventricle, the appropriate treatment is that of the underlying cause – in this case, hypertension. The aim in most patients is to control the blood pressure to a level below 140/90.

Commentary

There are many criteria for the ECG diagnosis of left ventricular hypertrophy, with varying sensitivity and specificity. Generally, the diagnostic criteria are quite specific (if the criteria are present, the likelihood of the patient having left ventricular hypertrophy is >90 per cent), but not very sensitive (the criteria will fail to detect 40–80 per cent of patients with left ventricular hypertrophy). The diagnostic criteria include:

- In the limb leads:
  - R wave greater than 11 mm in lead aVL
  - R wave greater than 20 mm in lead aVF
  - S wave greater than 14 mm in lead aVR
  - sum of R wave in lead I and S wave in lead III greater than 25 mm.
- In the chest leads:
  - R wave of 25 mm or more in the left chest leads
  - S wave of 25 mm or more in the right chest leads
  - sum of S wave in lead V_1 and R wave in lead V_5 or V_6 greater than 35 mm (Sokolow–Lyon criteria)
  - Sum of tallest R wave and deepest S wave in the chest leads greater than 45 mm.

- The **Cornell criteria** involve measuring S wave in lead V_3 and the R wave in lead aVL. Left ventricular hypertrophy is indicated by a sum of >28 mm in men and >20 mm in women.

- The **Romhilt–Estes scoring system** allocates points for the presence of certain criteria. A score of 5 indicates left ventricular hypertrophy and a score of 4 indicates probable left ventricular hypertrophy. Points are allocated as follows:
  - 3 points for (a) R or S wave in limb leads of 20 mm or more, (b) S wave in right chest leads of 25 mm or more, or (c) R wave in left chest leads of 25 mm or more
  - 3 points for ST segment and T wave changes ('typical strain') in a patient not taking digitalis (1 point with digitalis)
  - 3 points for P terminal force in V_1 greater than 1 mm deep with a duration greater than 0.04 s
  - 2 points for left axis deviation (beyond −15 degrees)
  - 1 point for QRS complex duration greater than 0.09 s
  - 1 point for intrinsicoid deflection (the interval from the start of the QRS complex to the peak of the R wave) in V_5 or V_6 greater than 0.05 s.

Further reading

Making Sense of the ECG: Left ventricular hypertrophy, p. 136.

CASE 36

Clinical scenario

Female, aged 79 years.

Presenting complaint

Breathlessness on exertion.

History of presenting complaint

Patient has had episodes of syncope and breathlessness for months. The syncope resolved following treatment but her breathlessness never improved back to normal. She now has episodes of paroxysmal nocturnal dyspnoea. As she attends the hospital regularly, she reported her persistent symptoms to the cardiac physiologist.

Past medical history

Congestive cardiac failure – unsure of medication but been on escalating doses of several drugs since she developed breathlessness.

Examination

Pulse: 72 bpm, regular.

Blood pressure: 126/98.

JVP: elevated by 2 cm.

Heart sounds: systolic murmur 3/6 in mitral area.

Chest auscultation: unremarkable.

Mild pitting ankle oedema.

Investigations

FBC: Hb 11.6, WCC 4.2, platelets 176.

U&E: Na 133, K 4.3, urea 8.5, creatinine 234.

Chest X-ray: marked cardiomegaly, fluid in horizontal fissure.

Echocardiogram: moderate mitral regurgitation into a moderately dilated left atrium. Left ventricular function severely impaired (ejection fraction 24 per cent).

Questions

1 What does this ECG show?
2 What is the mechanism of this?
3 What are the likely causes?
4 What are the key issues in managing this patient?

ECG analysis

Rate	72 bpm
Rhythm	Ventricular pacing
QRS axis	−48°
P waves	Occasionally visible
PR interval	N/A
QRS duration	Prolonged (194 ms)
T waves	Abnormal
QTc interval	Prolonged (540 ms)

Answers

1 There are occasional P waves visible between some (but not all) of the QRS complexes and occasional P waves can be seen deforming the ST segment. There is however no association between P waves and QRS complexes, indicating complete heart block. In addition, the QRS complexes are broad and preceded by a distinct 'spike' – this is **ventricular pacing**. The patient has had a VVI permanent pacemaker implanted for a diagnosis of complete heart block.

2 The 'spike' is an electrical discharge from a pacemaker, either temporary or permanent. In this case, a permanent single chamber or VVI (see coding schema below) pacemaker has been implanted to relieve symptoms of syncope. This paces the ventricle at a preset rate, in this case 72 bpm. If a ventricular contraction is sensed, the pacemaker is 'inhibited' – all the beats on this ECG are 'paced' beats.

3 The pacemaker has been implanted because of complete heart block due to failure of intrinsic pacemaker function. The rate of the escape rhythm of the ventricles of approximately 15–40 bpm is inadequate for most activities and causes fatigue, dizziness and syncope.

4 The pacemaker to be implanted must be chosen with care. Insertion of a VVI pacemaker when there are P waves may cause syncope due to 'pacemaker syndrome', when an atrial contraction against a closed tricuspid valve during systole may produce a wave of blood to flow retrogradely into the cerebral veins. Generally speaking, in an active individual, physiological pacing with a 'dual chamber' or DDD pacemaker will harness atrial contractility and timing to optimize cardiac function.

Commentary

- Pacemakers are described by pacing codes:

  - The first letter of the code identifies the chambers that can be paced (A – atrium, V – ventricle, D – dual)
  - The second letter of the code identifies the chambers that can be sensed (A – atrium, V – ventricle, D – dual)
  - The third letter of the code identifies what the pacemaker does if it detects intrinsic activity (I – inhibited, T – triggered, D – dual)
  - The fourth letter identifies rate-responsiveness (R) if present
  - The fifth letter identifies anti-tachycardia functions, if present (P – pacing, S – shock delivered, D – dual)

- The most commonly encountered pacemakers are:

  - VVI – a single lead pacemaker that senses ventricular activity; if no activity is detected, the pacemaker will take over cardiac rhythm by pacing the ventricle.

  - AAI – the pacemaker has a single lead, this time sensing atrial activity; if no activity is detected, the pacemaker paces the atrium.
  - DDD – there are pacemaker leads in both atrium and ventricle and so it senses activity in both chambers. It can pace atrium, ventricle or both sequentially.
  - AAIR, VVIR and DDDR – are rate-responsive varieties of the above. The pacemaker adjusts its pacing rate according to the patient's level of activity to mimic physiological response to exercise. Several parameters can monitor activity, including vibration through a piezo-electric crystal, respiration and blood temperature.

Further reading

Making Sense of the ECG: Pacemakers, p 222; Selection of a permanent pacemaker, p 226; Pacing and the ECG, p 227.

CASE 37

Speed: 25 mm/s   Limb: 10 mm/mV   Chest: 10 mm/mV

Figure adapted with permission from the BMJ Publishing Group (*Heart* 1986; **55**: 291–4).

Clinical scenario

Male, aged 34 years.

Presenting complaint
Rapid regular palpitations.

History of presenting complaint
Three-year history of episodic rapid regular palpitations. The current episode started suddenly 1 h prior to presentation.

Past medical history
Nil.

Examination
Pulse: 150 bpm, regular.
Blood pressure: 132/82.
JVP: normal.
Heart sounds: normal (tachycardic).
Chest auscultation: unremarkable.

Investigations
FBC: Hb 15.1, WCC 6.0, platelets 381.
U&E: Na 139, K 4.7, urea 4.9, creatinine 80.
Chest X-ray: normal heart size, clear lung fields.

Questions

1 What arrhythmia is seen in the initial part of this recording?
2 What drug is likely to have been administered at the time point indicated by the arrow?
3 What rhythm changes are seen subsequently?

ECG analysis

Rate	150 bpm (during AVNRT)
Rhythm	Initially AVNRT, followed by second-degree atrioventricular block (with some aberrant conduction and a ventricular ectopic beat), then junctional rhythm and finally sinus rhythm
QRS axis	Unable to assess (single lead)
P waves	Not visible during AVNRT (normal during sinus rhythm)
PR interval	Prolonged (220 ms) during sinus rhythm
QRS duration	Normal (80 ms) during AVNRT
T waves	Normal
QTc interval	Normal (398 ms) during sinus rhythm

Answers

1 The first part of the recording shows a regular narrow-complex tachycardia (150 bpm) with no visible P waves.

This is **atrioventricular nodal re-entry tachycardia** (AVNRT). Other possibilities include:

- atrioventricular re-entry tachycardia (AVRT), although in AVRT inverted P waves are often seen halfway between QRS complexes
- atrial flutter with 2:1 atrioventricular block, although one would normally expect to see evidence of flutter waves.

2 The drug administered is **adenosine**, which briefly blocks the atrioventricular node and terminates the arrhythmia. This rules out atrial flutter (adenosine would help reveal flutter waves but would not terminate atrial flutter).

3 As everything settles down after the termination of the AVNRT, a number of further rhythms are seen:

- initially there are three sinus beats, with broad QRS complexes indicating aberrant conduction
- next there is a ventricular ectopic beat
- next there is a brief period of 2:1 (second-degree) atrioventricular block, with alternate P waves not being conducted to the ventricles
- next there are five junctional beats (narrow complex, without a preceding P wave)

• finally the rhythm returns to normal sinus rhythm (100 bpm) with first-degree atrioventricular block (PR interval 220 ms).

The absence of a short PR interval or pre-excitation (delta wave) during sinus rhythm makes an accessory pathway unlikely, and thus makes the initial rhythm more likely to be AVNRT than AVRT.

Commentary

● The mechanism of AVNRT is discussed in Case 29.

● Given intravenously, adenosine transiently blocks the atrioventricular node. Adenosine is rapidly metabolized (half life 8–10 s) and therefore must be given quickly (over 2 s) into a central or large peripheral vein, followed by a flush of normal saline. Before giving adenosine, patients should be warned that they are likely to feel unwell for a few seconds, and may experience symptoms such as facial flushing and chest tightness. Adenosine is contraindicated in asthma, in second- or third-degree atrioventricular block and sick sinus syndrome (unless a pacemaker is fitted). Adenosine is potentiated by dipyridamole and so, if it is essential to give adenosine to someone taking dipyridamole, a much smaller dose

should be used. Patients with heart transplants can also be very sensitive to the effects of adenosine.

● Re-entry arrhythmias (AVRT and AVNRT) can be terminated by adenosine, as blocking the atrioventricular node breaks the re-entry circuit. In atrial flutter and fibrillation, blocking the atrioventricular node with adenosine will transiently slow atrioventricular nodal conduction and help reveal the underlying atrial activity – this can be useful diagnostically, but will not terminate the arrhythmia. In ventricular tachycardia, adenosine will have no effect (except in rare cases of fascicular ventricular tachycardia).

● AVNRT (and AVRT) can also be terminated with other atrioventricular nodal blocking manoeuvres, such as carotid sinus massage and the Valsalva manoeuvre.

Further reading
Making Sense of the ECG: Atrioventricular re-entry tachycardias, p 47.

Saito D, Ueeda M, Abe Y et al. Treatment of paroxysmal supraventricular tachycardia with intravenous injection of adenosine triphosphate. *Heart* 1986; **55**: 291–4.

CASE 38

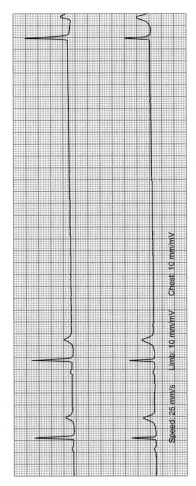

Speed: 25 mm/s   Limb: 10 mm/mV   Chest: 10 mm/mV

Clinical scenario

Male, aged 69 years.

Presenting complaint
Felt unwell while driving.

History of presenting complaint
Occasional episodes of dizziness. One episode of collapse and unconsciousness while driving resulted in admission following a road traffic accident.

Past medical history
Nil of note.

Examination
Pulse: 45 bpm with long pauses.
Blood pressure: 124/78.
JVP: not elevated.
Heart sounds: normal.
Chest auscultation: unremarkable.
No peripheral oedema.

Investigations
FBC: Hb 13.9, WCC 6.6, platelets 203.
U&E: Na 139, K 3.9, urea 5.0, creatinine 109.
Chest X-ray: normal heart size, clear lung fields.
Echocardiogram: structurally normal valves, normal left ventricular function.

Questions

1 What does this ECG show?
2 What is the mechanism of this?
3 What are the key issues in managing this patient?

ECG analysis

Rate	45 bpm, followed by a 5.2 s pause
Rhythm	Sinus bradycardia followed by sinus arrest, then a junctional escape beat
QRS axis	Unable to assess
P waves	Normal (when present)
PR interval	Borderline prolonged (200 ms)
QRS duration	Normal (80 ms)
T waves	Normal
QTc interval	Normal (420 ms)

Answers

1 This ECG rhythm strip shows two leads. There are two sinus beats, with a bradycardic heart rate of 45 bpm. There is then a pause of 5.2 s, during which no P waves are present. This is followed by a junctional escape beat. This is an episode of **sinus arrest**. The preceding sinus bradycardia is suggestive of underlying **sinus node dysfunction** (SND).

2 The sinus node fails to discharge reliably and 'on time' – there is cessation of P wave activity for a variable and unpredictable time period (compare this with sinoatrial node exit block – Case 20). It can also be caused by excessive vagal inhibition, infarction, fibrosis, acute myocarditis, cardiomyopathy, drugs (digoxin, procainamide, quinidine) or amyloidosis. A slower subsidiary pacemaker further down the conduction pathway will sometimes take over – in this case, the atrioventricular junction (as evidenced by a beat with a narrow QRS complex but no preceding P wave).

3 If asymptomatic, no treatment is required, although drugs that can disrupt sinus node function should be withdrawn. Symptoms include sudden onset of confusion, breathlessness, syncope, chest pain, fatigue, or, if the event occurs at night, disturbed sleep. Symptoms can be relieved by implanting a permanent pacemaker. An atrial (AAI) pacemaker monitors and paces the atrium. Some patients also demonstrate atrioventricular conduction problems and a dual chamber (DDD) pacemaker is necessary to restore atrioventricular sequential pacing.

Commentary

● Sinus arrest should be distinguished from sinoatrial node exit block. In sinus node arrest, the sinoatrial node stops firing for a *variable* time period, so the next P wave occurs after a *variable* interval. In sinoatrial node exit block there is a pause with one or more absent P waves, and then the next P wave appears exactly where predicted – in other words, the sinoatrial node continues to 'keep time', but its impulses are not transmitted beyond the node to the atria.

● Sinus arrest and sinoatrial node exit block can both be features of sinus node dysfunction (SND), formerly known as sick sinus syndrome. Other features of SND can include sinus bradycardia (as seen here), brady-tachy syndrome and atrial fibrillation.

● Patients who drive a vehicle and who suffer from pre-syncope or syncope should receive appropriate advice about driving – very often, they will be barred from driving until the problem has been diagnosed and/or corrected as appropriate. Driving regulations vary between countries. In the UK, information on the medical aspects of fitness to drive can be found on the website of Driver and Vehicle Licensing Agency (www.dvla.gov.uk).

Further reading
Making Sense of the ECG: Sinus bradycardia, p 31; Sinus arrest, p 35; Sinoatrial block, p 36.

CASE 39

LOC: 00000 – 0000   Speed: 25 mm/sec   Limb: 10 mm/mV   Chest: 10 mm/mV

50~ 0.15–150 Hz

15726

Clinical scenario

Male, aged 24 years.

Presenting complaint
Routine ECG for insurance medical.

History of presenting complaint
No history – normally fit and well.

Past medical history
No prior medical history.

Examination
Pulse: 66 bpm, regular.
Blood pressure: 120/74.
JVP: not elevated.
Heart sounds: normal.
Chest auscultation: unremarkable.
No peripheral oedema.

Investigations
FBC: Hb 13.8, WCC 5.1, platelets 345.
U&E: Na 143, K 4.8, urea 4.7, creatinine 68.
Chest X-ray: normal heart size, clear lung fields.

Questions

1   What does this ECG show?
2   What should you do next?

ECG analysis

Rate	66 bpm
Rhythm	Sinus rhythm
QRS axis	Right axis deviation (+152°)
P waves	Inverted in leads I and aVL, biphasic in lead aVR
PR interval	Normal (160 ms)
QRS duration	Normal (70 ms)
T waves	Inverted in leads I and aVL, upright in lead aVR
QTc interval	Normal (420 ms)

Answers

1 This ECG has an unusual appearance:

• There is extreme right axis deviation (+152°), and a positive QRS complex in lead aVR.

• The QRS complexes in leads I and aVL are negative, and there is P wave and T wave inversion in these leads too. These appearances are difficult to account for clinically – although similar appearances are seen in the limb leads in dextrocardia, we would also expect to find abnormalities in the chest leads in dextrocardia (whereas in this patient the chest leads are normal). Moreover, the patient's clinical examination and chest X-ray have not shown dextrocardia. This patient's ECG appearances are therefore due to **misplacement of the right and left arm electrodes.**

2 Check the ECG electrode positioning and reposition the right and left arm electrodes on the appropriate limb, so that the ECG can be repeated with all the electrodes in the correct place. When this patient's ECG was repeated, with the arm electrodes positioned correctly, it was found to be normal.

Commentary

● It is thought that errors in electrode placement are made in up to 4 per cent of ECG recordings. When recording an ECG it is essential to check the electrode positioning carefully, as electrode misplacement can cause significant changes in the ECG's appearance and therefore lead to diagnosis (and treatment) errors.

● Any permutation of the limb and chest electrodes is theoretically possible, but the commonest electrode placement errors involve switching two of the limb electrodes or two of the chest electrodes.

● ECGs should always be assessed in the patient's clinical context, and ECG abnormalities that are unexpected or 'don't make sense' should always prompt a check of whether the ECG was recorded correctly.

● When an electrode placement error is recognized, the ECG should be repeated (with correct electrode placement) at the earliest opportunity.

Further reading

Making Sense of the ECG: How do I record an ECG? p 16; Electrode misplacement, p 217.

Rudiger A, Hellermann JP, Mukherjee R *et al.* Electrocardiographic artifacts due to electrode misplacement and their frequency in different clinical settings. *Am J Emerg Med* 2007; **25**: 174–8.

CASE 40

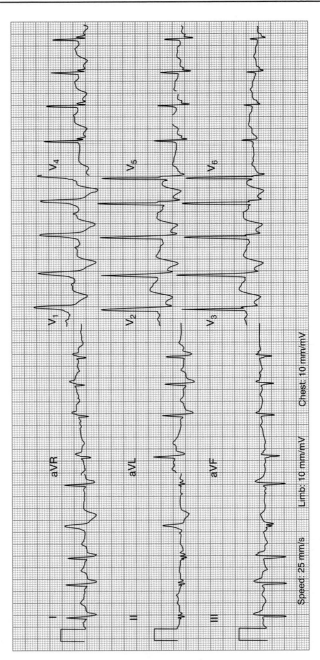

Speed: 25 mm/s   Limb: 10 mm/mV   Chest: 10 mm/mV

Clinical scenario

Female, aged 81 years.

Presenting complaint
Severe central chest pain.

History of presenting complaint
Patient was walking to local shops. Experienced rapid onset of severe central crushing chest pain, associated with breathlessness and nausea. Similar to (but much worse than) her usual angina.

Past medical history
Exertional angina for many years.
Mild hypertension.
Type 2 diabetes mellitus.

Examination
Pulse: 108 bpm, regular with occasional ectopic beats.
Blood pressure: 108/76.

JVP: not elevated.
Heart sounds: normal.
Chest auscultation: unremarkable.
No peripheral oedema.

Investigations
FBC: Hb 12.1, WCC 4.7, platelets 390.
U&E: Na 141, K 4.9, urea 5.1, creatinine 143.
Troponin I: elevated at 28.6 (after 12 h).
Chest X-ray: mild cardiomegaly.
Echocardiogram: trace of mitral regurgitation but valve structurally normal. Left ventricle mildly impaired (ejection fraction 52 per cent), with posterior wall hypokinesia.

Questions

1 What does this ECG show?
2 What is the mechanism of this?
3 What treatment would be appropriate in this patient?

ECG analysis

Rate	108 bpm
Rhythm	Sinus rhythm with occasional ventricular ectopic beats
QRS axis	Left axis deviation (+36°)
P waves	Normal
PR interval	Normal (160 ms)
QRS duration	Upper limit of normal (120 ms)
T waves	Limb leads normal. Chest leads – merged with ST segment
QTc interval	Prolonged (480 ms)

Additional comments

There are tall dominant R waves in leads V_1–V_4 with ST segment depression.

Answers

1 This ECG shows tall dominant R waves in leads with ST segment depression in the anterior chest leads. This is an **acute posterior ST elevation myocardial infarction (STEMI)**.

2 Posterior STEMI results from occlusion of the coronary artery supplying the posterior wall of the heart – in 70 per cent of cases, the right coronary artery (and in the remainder the circumflex artery).

3 Aspirin 300 mg orally (then 75 mg once daily), clopidogrel 300 mg orally (then 75 mg once daily for one month), glyceryl trinitrate sublingually, pain relief (diamorphine, plus an anti-emetic), oxygen. Prompt restoration of myocardial blood flow is required, either through primary percutaneous coronary intervention (PCI) or, if primary PCI is not available, thrombolysis.

Commentary

● On a conventional ECG, the usual STEMI appearances of pathological Q waves, ST segment elevation and inverted T waves will, in a posterior STEMI, be seen as *reciprocal* changes in the anterior leads V_1–V_3, i.e. *R waves* (instead of Q waves), ST segment *depression* (instead of elevation) and *upright* T waves (rather than inverted) when viewed from leads V_1–V_3.

● The hallmark ST segment elevation of an acute STEMI is not seen in an acute posterior myocardial infarction unless an ECG is recorded using posterior leads, V_7–V_9, on the back of the chest. Posterior myocardial infarctions are therefore commonly overlooked, or misdiagnosed as anterior wall ischaemia. Using posterior leads helps to distinguish between the two diagnoses.

● In the clinical context of acute chest pain with ST segment depression in the anterior or antero-septal leads, always consider the possibility of posterior myocardial infarction.

● Posterior myocardial infarction is one cause of a 'dominant' R wave in lead V_1. Other causes are:
  ● right ventricular hypertrophy
  ● Wolff–Parkinson–White syndrome with a left-sided accessory pathway.

Further reading

Making Sense of the ECG: Posterior myocardial infarction, p 139; Acute posterior myocardial infarction, p 179.

CASE 41

Speed: 25 mm/s   Limb: 10 mm/mV   Chest: 10 mm/mV

Clinical scenario

Female, aged 83 years.

Presenting complaint
Found collapsed at home.

History of presenting complaint
Patient found lying on the floor of her home by a
neighbour. She had slipped and fallen the previous
evening when preparing to go to bed, and was found
11 h later having been on the floor all night. She had
fractured her right hip and was unable to stand.

Past medical history
Stroke 4 years earlier (full recovery).

Examination
Reduced conscious level (Glasgow Coma Scale score
11/15).

Right leg shortened and externally rotated.

Temperature: 30.8°C.
Pulse: 96 bpm, irregularly irregular.
Blood pressure: 98/54.
JVP: not elevated.
Heart sounds: normal.
Chest auscultation: unremarkable.
No peripheral oedema.

Investigations
FBC: Hb 11.8, WCC 17.1, platelets 182.
U&E: Na 134, K 5.1, urea 11.7, creatinine 148.
Chest X-ray: normal heart size, clear lung fields.
Creatine kinase: elevated at 1565.

Questions

1 What does this ECG show?
2 What is the cause of these ECG appearances?
3 What other ECG findings may be seen in this condition?
4 What treatment is indicated?

ECG analysis

Rate	96 bpm
Rhythm	Atrial fibrillation
QRS axis	Right axis deviation (+98°)
P waves	Absent (atrial fibrillation)
PR interval	Not applicable
QRS duration	Normal (90 ms)
T waves	Normal
QTc interval	Prolonged (472 ms)

Additional comments

J waves (also known as 'Osborn waves') are visible in lead V_4.

Answers

1 This ECG shows atrial fibrillation with J waves, also known as Osborn waves. The J wave is a small positive deflection seen at the junction between the QRS complex and the ST segment and is usually best seen in the inferior limb leads and the lateral chest leads (in this case the J waves are most clearly seen in lead V_4). The corrected QT interval is prolonged at 472 ms.

2 Hypothermia (the patient's temperature is 30.8°C).

3 J waves, atrial fibrillation and prolongation of the QT interval are all features of hypothermia. In addition, the ECG in hypothermia may also show broadening of the QRS complexes, lengthening of the PR interval, atrioventricular block, ventricular arrhythmias and asystole.

4 The treatment of hypothermia includes gradual rewarming and the administration, where appropriate, of warm intravenous fluids and warm humidified oxygen. Careful monitoring of vital signs and of the ECG is required. Passive rewarming is suitable for most patients with mild hypothermia; active rewarming should be considered for those with moderate or severe hypothermia. Co-morbidities (e.g. sepsis or, in this case, a hip fracture) should be managed appropriately.

Commentary

● J waves, also known as Osborn waves, are characterized by a dome- or hump-shaped deflection of the ECG at the junction of the QRS complex and the ST segment (the J point). J waves have been reported to be present in around 80 per cent of ECGs in hypothermic patients (below 33°C), but they are also sometimes seen in patients with a normal body temperature and are therefore not completely specific for hypothermia.

● A variety of arrhythmias can be seen in hypothermia. Sinus tachycardia is the earliest abnormality, followed (as core temperature falls) by sinus bradycardia, then atrial ectopics and atrial fibrillation (often with a slow ventricular rate). As the temperature falls further, the QRS complexes become increasingly broad and the risk of ventricular fibrillation increases. Finally, asystole occurs.

● Ventricular fibrillation can be refractory to defibrillation in the severely hypothermic patient. In patients with a core temperature below 30°C, the onset of

ventricular tachycardia or fibrillation should be treated with an attempt at defibrillation – if this is ineffective, further attempts should be deferred until the patient's core temperature is above 30°C. The use of drugs such as adrenaline and lidocaine is not recommended at a core temperature below 30°C, as they are usually ineffective and can accumulate in the circulation, only to be released later at toxic levels as the patient rewarms.

Further reading

Making Sense of the ECG: Are J waves present? p 183.
Epstein E, Anna K. Accidental hypothermia. *BMJ* 2006; **332**: 706–9.
Mattu A, Brady W, Perron A. Electrocardiographic manifestations of hypothermia. *Am J Emerg Med* 2002; **20**: 314–26.

CASE 42

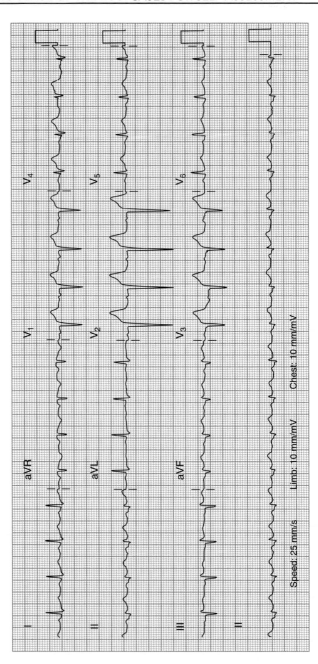

Clinical scenario

Male, aged 65 years.

Presenting complaint
Breathlessness on exertion, but no chest pain.

History of presenting complaint
Patient had a heart attack 6 months previously (thrombolysed). Never returned to previous activity levels. In past few weeks, noticed more breathlessness than usual – had to avoid stairs as much as possible, and steep paths were now impossible. Occasional paroxysmal nocturnal dyspnoea. Patient had a similar ECG in his wallet, given to him on discharge from previous admission.

Past medical history
No history of lung disease.

Examination
Pulse: 96 bpm, regular.
Blood pressure: 114/66.
JVP: not elevated.
Heart sounds: normal.
Chest auscultation: bilateral inspiratory crackles.
No peripheral oedema.

Investigations
FBC: Hb 12.7, WCC 8.0, platelets 284.
U&E: Na 139, K 4.6, urea 4.8, creatinine 124.
Troponin I: negative.
Chest X-ray: enlarged left ventricle. Pulmonary oedema.
Echocardiogram: awaited.

Questions

1 What does this ECG show?
2 What would be the most useful investigation?
3 What are the key issues in managing this patient?

ECG analysis

Rate	96 bpm
Rhythm	Sinus rhythm
QRS axis	Normal ($-10°$)
P waves	Normal
PR interval	Normal (160 ms)
QRS duration	Normal (100 ms)
T waves	Normal
QTc interval	Mildly prolonged (455 ms)

Additional comments

There are deep anterior Q waves with persistent ST segment elevation.

Answers

1 Deep Q waves with persistent ST segment elevation in leads V_1–V_4, six months after a previous myocardial infarction, is suggestive of a **left ventricular aneurysm.**

2 An echocardiogram would confirm the presence of a left ventricular aneurysm and allow assessment of left ventricular function and any valvular dysfunction. A cardiac magnetic resonance scan is also useful for delineating the extent of any aneurysmal segment and also assessing myocardial viability.

3 Although the ST segment elevation on the admission ECG may suggest a new infarction, the history (progressive breathlessness without chest pain) is not compatible with this diagnosis. A chest X-ray will show an abnormal silhouette and the troponin level will be in the normal range. Comparison with a pre-discharge ECG from the time of his previous infarction allows confirmation that the ST segment elevation is longstanding. Patients may present with heart failure, an embolic event, intractable arrhythmias or chest pain. Treatment of heart failure, rhythm abnormalities and anticoagulation are required as appropriate. Surgical resection of the aneurysm (aneurysmectomy) with or without endocardial patching may improve symptoms.

Commentary

● Coronary artery disease and acute myocardial infarction are the most common causes of a left ventricular aneurysm. Rarer causes include trauma, Chagas' disease and sarcoidosis.

● Left ventricular aneurysm is a late complication of myocardial infarction, seen in around 10 per cent of survivors.

● Left ventricular aneurysm may present as:

● breathlessness – aneurysmal tissue is non-contractile, so an extensive aneurysm may cause loss of a large proportion of left ventricular function and lead to symptoms and signs of heart failure

● ventricular arrhythmia – the ischaemic border zone is a substrate for ventricular extrasystoles and ventricular tachycardia

● sudden death – due to ventricular arrhythmias, or to spontaneous rupture of the aneurysmal segment

● chest pain – the border zone between infarcted aneurysmal tissue and healthy, non-infarcted myocardium can become ischaemic

● embolism – thrombus may form in a ventricular aneurysm, due to relative stasis of blood, and embolize.

Further reading

Making Sense of the ECG: Are the ST segments elevated? p 159; Left ventricular aneurysm, p 169.

CASE 43

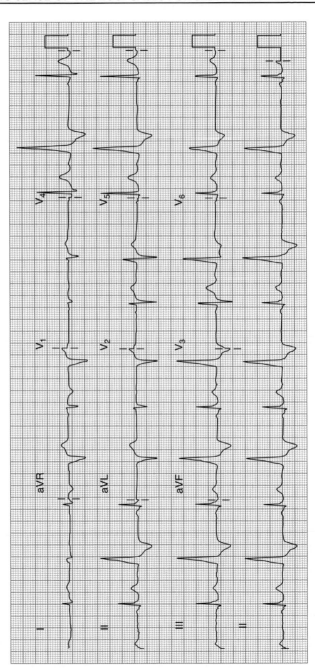

Clinical scenario

Male, aged 78 years.

Presenting complaint
Asymptomatic.

History of presenting complaint
Patient attended for preoperative screening for a right inguinal hernia repair. His pulse was noted to be irregular, and this ECG was performed.

Past medical history
Right inguinal hernia. No prior cardiovascular history.

Examination
Pulse: 66 bpm, regularly irregular.
Blood pressure: 134/76.
JVP: not elevated.
Heart sounds: regularly irregular.
Chest auscultation: unremarkable.
No peripheral oedema.

Investigations
FBC: Hb 13.5, WCC 6.1, platelets 318.
U&E: Na 137, K 4.2, urea 4.8, creatinine 80.
Thyroid function: normal.
Chest X-ray: normal heart size, clear lung fields.
Echocardiogram: normal cardiac structure and function.

Questions

1 What arrhythmia does this ECG show?
2 Where in the heart has this arrhythmia originated?

ECG analysis

Rate	66 bpm
Rhythm	Ventricular bigeminy
QRS axis	Normal (+80°) for sinus beats, inferior axis for ventricular ectopic beats
P waves	Present for sinus beats
PR interval	160 ms
QRS duration	Normal (80 ms) for sinus beats, broad (140 ms) for ventricular ectopic beats
T waves	Normal for sinus beats, inverted for ventricular ectopic beats
QTc interval	Normal (440 ms)

Answers

1 In this ECG every normal sinus beat is followed by a broad and abnormally shaped QRS complex, a ventricular ectopic beat (VEB). This 1:1 coupling between sinus beats and VEBs is called **ventricular bigeminy**.

2 As the name suggests, VEBs arise within the ventricles. In this case the VEBs have a left bundle branch block morphology in the chest leads, indicating an origin in the right ventricle. The VEBs also have an inferior axis in the limb leads (positive complexes in leads II, III and aVF) indicating an origin in the superior part of the ventricle. Taken together, these features suggest the most likely origin of the VEBs is in the upper right ventricle, most probably the right ventricular outflow tract.

Commentary

● An ectopic beat arises earlier than the next normal (sinus) beat would have occurred (in contrast to escape beats, which arise later than expected).

● Ventricular ectopic beats cause broad QRS complexes (unlike supraventricular ectopics, which usually cause narrow QRS complexes). The ventricular ectopic impulse, having arisen within the ventricular myocardium, has to conduct from myocyte to myocyte in order to depolarize the ventricles – this is slower than conduction via the His–Purkinje system, and hence ventricular depolarization takes longer than it would with a normal sinus beat.

● VEBs arising from the right ventricle have a left bundle branch block morphology, and those arising from the left ventricle have a right bundle branch block morphology.

● On checking the radial pulse of a patient with bigeminy, the VEBs usually feel weaker than the normal sinus beats (because the ventricle has not filled fully by the time systole occurs). The normal sinus beat after the VEB can also feel stronger than usual, as there will have been a slightly longer period for ventricular filling due to the compensatory pause after the VEB ('extrasystolic potentiation'). As a result, VEBs may sometimes be missed on palpation of the radial pulse. Patients with ventricular bigeminy are therefore sometimes mistakenly diagnosed as being bradycardic when their pulse is taken at the wrist, if only the sinus beats are counted. Even automated monitoring equipment (e.g. blood pressure monitors, pulse oximeters) can sometimes underestimate the heart rate by 'missing' the VEBs. Careful inspection of an ECG will reveal the correct heart rate.

● For more information on the investigation and management of VEBs, see the commentary on Case 9.

Further reading

Making Sense of the ECG: Ectopic beats, p 61.
Ng GA. Treating patients with ventricular ectopic beats. *Heart* 2006; **92**: 1707–12.

CASE 44

Speed: 25 mm/s   Limb: 10 mm/mV   Chest: 10 mm/mV

Clinical scenario

Male, aged 26 years.

Presenting complaint
Breathlessness. Persistent nocturnal cough. Dizziness.

History of presenting complaint
Had been fit and well until 2 months ago when he had
a viral infection. Never really regained fitness
afterwards. Had had several courses of antibiotics from
family doctor but his symptoms persisted. Frequent
nocturnal waking with breathlessness. Became worried
when he found he was breathless walking around his
flat and he noticed his pulse was very erratic.

Past medical history
Nil else of note.
Smokes 10 cigarettes per day.
Drinks 12 units alcohol per week.
No family history of heart disease.

Examination
Pulse: 116 bpm, irregular.
Blood pressure: 118/88.
JVP: elevated by 4 cm.
Heart sounds: normal.
Chest auscultation: bi-basal crackles.
Pitting peripheral oedema to mid-calf.

Investigations
FBC: Hb 12.2, WCC 8.1, platelets 346.
U&E: Na 136, K 4.9, urea 7.8, creatinine 124.
Thyroid function: normal.
Troponin I: negative.
Chest X-ray: enlarged left ventricle. Pulmonary
oedema.
Echocardiogram: Dilated left ventricle with poor
function. Mildly impaired right ventricular function.
Functional mitral regurgitation.

Questions

1 What does this ECG show?
2 What is the likely cause?
3 What are the key issues in managing this patient?

ECG analysis

Rate	108 bpm overall, but very variable
Rhythm	Underlying sinus rhythm with frequent bursts of non-sustained ventricular tachycardia
QRS axis	Normal (+45°) in sinus rhythm, extreme axis deviation in VT
P waves	Normal
PR interval	Normal (172 ms)
QRS duration	Normal (90 ms) in sinus rhythm, broad complexes in ventricular tachycardia
T waves	Normal morphology where seen
QTc interval	Difficult to assess

Answers

1 Underlying sinus rhythm is seen with normal axis. There are frequent runs of non-sustained broad complex tachycardia with marked change in axis. These are bursts of **ventricular tachycardia.**

2 The underlying diagnosis is most likely to be a dilated cardiomyopathy secondary to viral myocarditis.

3 Treatment is aimed at controlling the signs and symptoms of congestive cardiac failure until resolution occurs – this may take weeks or months (if at all). Patients usually respond to a combination of loop diuretic, angiotensin-converting enzyme (ACE) inhibitor (titrated to the maximum tolerated dose while monitoring renal function), beta blocker (in escalating dose). Failure to respond to treatment warrants full investigation. Anti-arrhythmic drugs may be needed for ventricular tachyarrhythmias, and an implantable cardioverter-defibrillator (ICD) may be required for patients at high risk of cardiac arrest. Surgical options include a left ventricular assist device (LVAD) to support the function of the failing heart, and cardiac transplantation for those with severe heart failure that fails to improve.

Commentary

● Broad-complex tachycardia is due to ventricular tachycardia, or to supraventricular tachycardia (SVT) with aberrant conduction (such as bundle branch block or pre-excitation). Where there is doubt about the diagnosis, it should be assumed to be ventricular tachycardia until proven otherwise.

● Several ECG features can suggest ventricular tachycardia rather than SVT with aberrant conduction. These include:

● extreme axis deviation
● concordance of the QRS axis across the chest leads
● unusual QRS complexes that do not have a classical left or right bundle branch block appearance.

● Evidence of independent atrial activity is a virtually diagnostic feature of VT, although it is found in fewer than half of cases. Independent atrial activity is indicated by:

● independent P wave activity
● capture beats
● fusion beats.

● Dilated cardiomyopathy is the common expression of myocardial damage following a variety of insults. Viral infection, excess alcohol consumption or cytotoxic drugs are the most common causes but in many cases no cause is identified.

● At least two dozen viruses have been implicated as a cause of viral myocarditis. The commonest is Coxsackie with both A and B varieties able to damage the myocardium. This infection is often self-limiting and may be subclinical. Most patients recover within a few weeks, but some take months before symptoms resolve and ventricular function normalizes. Occasionally it is fatal.

Further reading

Making Sense of the ECG: Ventricular tachycardia, p 53; How do I distinguish between VT and SVT? p 74.
Wellens HJJ. Ventricular tachycardia: diagnosis of broad QRS complex tachycardia. 2001; *Heart* **86**: 579–85.

CASE 45

Speed: 25 mm/s   Limb: 10 mm/mV   Chest: 10 mm/mV

Clinical scenario

Male, aged 25 years.

Presenting complaint
Central chest pain, exacerbated by lying supine and on deep inspiration.

History of presenting complaint
Viral symptoms for 1 week, with chest pain for 3 days.

Past medical history
Nil.

Examination
Patient in discomfort and sitting upright.
Temperature: 38.1°C.

Pulse: 110 bpm, regular.
Blood pressure: 128/80.
JVP: not elevated.
Heart sounds: soft pericardial friction rub.
Chest auscultation: unremarkable.
No peripheral oedema.

Investigations
FBC: Hb 15.2, WCC 9.2, platelets 364.
U&E: Na 141, K 4.4, urea 3.8, creatinine 58.
ESR and CRP: elevated.
Thyroid function tests: normal.
Chest X-ray: normal heart size, clear lung fields.

Questions

1 What does the ECG show?
2 What other tests would be appropriate?
3 What can cause this condition?
4 What are the treatment options?

ECG analysis

Rate	110 bpm
Rhythm	Sinus rhythm
QRS axis	Normal (+65°)
P waves	Normal
PR interval	Normal (160 ms)
QRS duration	Normal (80 ms)
T waves	Normal
QTc interval	Normal (433 ms)

Additional comments

There is widespread ST segment elevation (concave upward or 'saddle-shaped') in leads I, II, III, aVF and V_2–V_6, with reciprocal ST segment depression in lead aVR.

Answers

1 This ECG shows widespread ST segment elevation (concave upward or 'saddle-shaped') in leads I, II, III, aVF and V_2–V_6, with reciprocal ST segment depression in lead aVR. In the clinical context, these findings are consistent with a diagnosis of pericarditis.

2 In addition to those listed, other appropriate tests would include:

• cardiac markers (troponins, creatine kinase)
• echocardiography
• viral serology with or without other microbiology as indicated
• autoantibody screen, complement levels, immuno-globulins.

3 Pericarditis has many causes, including:

• idiopathic
• infective (viral, bacterial, tuberculous, fungal, parasitic)
• myocardial infarction (first few days)
• Dressler's syndrome (1 month or more post-myocardial infarction)
• uraemia
• malignancy
• connective tissue disease
• radiotherapy
• traumatic
• drug-induced.

4 Direct treatment of the underlying cause is important where applicable. Anti-inflammatory drugs (e.g. aspirin, indometacin) can be effective. Steroids can be considered in selected cases, but their use is controversial and specialist advice should be sought. Colchicine can be useful in the management of relapsing pericarditis.

Commentary

● The ST segment elevation of pericarditis is typically widespread, appearing in more leads than one would normally expect for an acute myocardial infarction. The morphology of the ST segment elevation is described as concave upwards or 'saddle shaped'. As the pericarditis settles, the ST segments gradually return to baseline and, in the longer term, there may be residual T wave inversion.

● Patients with pericarditis and ST segment elevation will often have an elevation in their cardiac markers (troponins and creatine kinase) as a result of a degree of coexistent myocarditis. It is important not to misdiagnose acute myocardial infarction, and a coronary angiogram may be required to clarify the diagnosis.

● Echocardiography is important to monitor for the appearance of a pericardial effusion (not always present, but may develop as a complication). This can cause cardiac tamponade.

● The differential diagnosis of ST segment elevation includes acute myocardial infarction, left ventricular aneurysm, Prinzmetal's (vasospastic) angina, pericarditis, high take-off, left bundle branch block and Brugada syndrome.

Further reading

Making Sense of the ECG: Are the ST segments elevated? p 159; Pericarditis, p 172.
Oakley CM. Myocarditis, pericarditis and other pericardial diseases. *Heart* 2000; **84**: 449–54.

CASE 46

Speed: 25 mm/s   Limb: 10 mm/mV   Chest: 10 mm/mV

Figure adapted with permission from the BMJ Publishing Group (*Heart* 2007, **93**, 1630–6).

Clinical scenario

Male, aged 76 years.

Presenting complaint
Asymptomatic (incidental finding).

History of presenting complaint
Presented to family doctor for a routine health check.

Past medical history
Nil of note.

Examination
Pulse: 156 bpm, regular.
Blood pressure: 116/90.
JVP: not elevated.

Heart sounds: normal.
Chest auscultation: unremarkable.
No peripheral oedema.

Investigations
FBC: Hb 13.8, WCC 5.3, platelets 243.
U&E: Na 137, K 4.8, urea 5.9, creatinine 107.
Thyroid function: normal.
Troponin I: negative.
Chest X-ray: normal heart size, clear lung fields.
Echocardiogram: normal valves. Good left ventricular
function (ejection fraction 63 per cent).

Questions

1 What rhythm does this ECG show?
2 What treatment has been given during the recording?
3 What are the key issues in managing this patient?

ECG analysis

Rate	156 bpm
Rhythm	Atrial flutter
QRS axis	Normal (+74°)
P waves	Not visible (flutter waves are present)
PR interval	N/A
QRS duration	Normal (70 ms)
T waves	Not clearly visible
QTc interval	Normal (406 ms)

Answers

1 There are no P waves visible on this 12-lead ECG but there are low amplitude flutter waves at around 300/min which give a 'saw-tooth' baseline: this is **atrial flutter**. As is commonly the case with atrial flutter, there is 2:1 atrioventricular block (in the first part of the recording) giving rise to a ventricular rate of around 150 bpm.

2 Towards the right of the ECG trace, the QRS complexes disappear and all we see are the flutter waves.

This is **atrioventricular block induced by adenosine**, which can be helpful diagnostically in revealing the underlying atrial rhythm by transiently blocking the atrioventricular node and thereby blocking ventricular activity for a few seconds. Similar atrioventricular block can be achieved with carotid sinus massage. Adenosine will not terminate atrial flutter, but it can terminate arrhythmias where the re-entry circuit involves the atrioventricular node (AVRT and AVNRT).

3 The causes of atrial flutter are the same as atrial fibrillation, namely coronary artery, hypertensive and rheumatic heart disease, hyperthyroidism, dilated and hypertrophic cardiomyopathy, sick sinus syndrome, cardiac and thoracic surgery, alcohol misuse (acute and chronic), constrictive pericarditis and idiopathic. The aims of treatment are:

- ventricular rate control, as with atrial fibrillation
- anticoagulation where appropriate
- to terminate the atrial flutter pharmacologically, by electrical cardioversion or by an atrial flutter ablation procedure.

Commentary

● Atrial flutter can be difficult to diagnose if the 'saw-tooth' pattern of the flutter waves is not clearly seen. Blocking the atrioventricular node briefly will not terminate the arrhythmia, but it will help reveal the underlying atrial rhythm. The node can be blocked with adenosine, or by performing carotid sinus massage.

● Given intravenously, adenosine transiently blocks the atrioventricular node. Adenosine is rapidly metabolized (half life 8–10 s) and therefore must be given quickly (over 2 s) into a central or large peripheral vein, followed by a flush of normal saline. Before giving adenosine, patients should be warned that they are likely to feel unwell for a few seconds, and may experience symptoms such as facial flushing and chest tightness. Adenosine is contraindicated in asthma, in second- or third-degree atrioventricular block and sick sinus syndrome (unless a pacemaker is fitted). Adenosine is potentiated by dipyridamole and so, if it is essential to give adenosine to someone taking dipyridamole, a much smaller dose should be used. Patients with heart transplants can also be very sensitive to the effects of adenosine.

● Controlling the ventricular rate with medication can be difficult. Options include beta blockers, verapamil, digoxin and amiodarone.

● Sinus rhythm can be restored with DC cardioversion. Pharmacological options for restoring (and maintaining) sinus rhythm include sotalol, flecainide and amiodarone. However, these drugs don't always work.

● An atrial flutter ablation procedure is also an effective, albeit invasive, treatment option.

Further reading

Making Sense of the ECG: Atrial flutter, p 39.

CASE 47

Speed: 25 mm/s   Limb: 10 mm/mV   Chest: 10 mm/mV

Clinical scenario

Female, aged 63 years.

Presenting complaint
Asymptomatic – routine ECG performed at follow-up visit to cardiology outpatient clinic.

History of presenting complaint
Nil – patient currently asymptomatic.

Past medical history
Treated for sick sinus syndrome 2 years ago.

Examination
Pulse: 70 bpm, regular.
Blood pressure: 138/78.
JVP: not elevated.
Heart sounds: normal.
Chest auscultation: unremarkable.
No peripheral oedema.

Investigations
FBC: Hb 13.8, WCC 5.7, platelets 240.
U&E: Na 141, K 4.3, urea 2.8, creatinine 68.

Questions

1 What does this ECG show?
2 What device did this patient receive 2 years ago to treat their sick sinus syndrome?
3 Does this device have one electrode or two? How might you find out?
4 What do you understand by the term AAIR?

ECG analysis

Rate	70 bpm
Rhythm	Atrial pacing
QRS axis	–
P waves	Present following atrial pacing spike
PR interval	Short
QRS duration	Normal (80 ms)
T waves	Biphasic (initially positive but with negative terminal deflection)
QTc interval	Normal (350 ms)

Additional comments

Pacing spikes are evident prior to each P wave.

Answers

1 There are sharp downward vertical deflections prior to each P wave. These represent pacing spikes. The position of these prior to the P wave indicates atrial pacing.

2 The patient has had a pacemaker implanted 2 years ago to treat their sick sinus syndrome. The tip of the atrial pacemaker lead is probably located close to the atrioventricular node, as atrial activation occurs close to ventricular activation (short PR interval).

3 It is not possible to say. The pacemaker is certainly capable of pacing the atria, as evidenced by pacing spikes followed by P waves, and an atrial pacing electrode must therefore be present. However, the absence of ventricular pacing does not rule out the possibility that a ventricular electrode is also present – if it is a dual chamber pacemaker, the ventricular lead may simply be monitoring ventricular activity but not supplying any pacing spikes at present. If in doubt, most patients with pacemakers will carry a pacemaker identity card. Failing that, a chest X-ray will reveal the number of pacing electrodes. This patient actually had a single chamber pacemaker (AAIR).

4 The term AAIR is a pacing code, and describes a pacemaker that paces the atrium, senses the atrium, is inhibited by intrinsic atrial activity, and is rate-responsive.

CASE 47 189

Commentary

● Permanent pacemakers can be single chamber (a single electrode pacing/sensing either the right atrium or the right ventricle) or dual chamber (two electrodes, one to pace/sense the right atrium and another to pace/sense to right ventricle).

● For sick sinus syndrome, a single chamber atrial pacemaker is usually appropriate unless there are any problems (or potential problems) with atrioventricular node conduction, in which case a dual chamber pacemaker is a better option.

● Pacemakers can be identified on the ECG by their pacing spikes. The presence of a pacing spike followed by a P wave indicates atrial pacing. A pacing spike followed by a QRS complex indicates ventricular pacing.

● Pacemakers are described by pacing codes:

● The first letter of the code identifies the chambers that can be paced (A – atrium, V – ventricle, D – dual).

● The second letter of the code identifies the chambers that can be sensed (A – atrium, V – ventricle, D – dual).

● The third letter of the code identifies what the pacemaker does if it detects intrinsic activity (I – inhibited, T – triggered, D – dual).

● The fourth letter identifies rate-responsiveness (R) if present.

● The fifth letter identifies anti-tachycardia functions, if present (P – pacing, S – shock delivered, D – dual).

Thus an AAIR pacemaker can pace the atrium. However, if it senses intrinsic atrial activity (normal P waves), it will be inhibited and stop pacing. The R indicates that it is rate-responsive, and can therefore increase its pacing rate (and thus the patient's heart rate) if it detects that the patient is undertaking physical exertion. Pacemakers can detect physical activity by monitoring a variety of indicators including vibration, respiration or blood temperature.

Further reading
Making Sense of the ECG: Sick sinus syndrome, p 35; Pacing and the ECG, p 227.
Morgan JM. 2006. Basics of cardiac pacing: selection and mode choice. *Heart* **92**, 850–54.

CASE 48

Clinical Scenario

Female, aged 84 years.

Presenting complaint

Felt dizzy then collapsed in nursing home.

History of presenting complaint

Nursing home staff reported that this previously very active woman had not been her usual self for a few days, with dizziness especially on standing. The doctor who was called to see her recorded that her pulse was very slow.

Past medical history

Type 2 diabetes mellitus.
Rheumatoid disease.
Mild heart failure.

Examination

Pulse: 43 bpm, regular.
Blood pressure: 122/76.
JVP: cannon waves visible.
Heart sounds: soft systolic murmur in aortic area.
Chest auscultation: unremarkable.
Trace of pitting ankle oedema.

Investigations

FBC: Hb 10.3, WCC 4.9, platelets 189.
U&E: Na 135, K 3.2, urea 6.8, creatinine 176.
Thyroid function: normal.
Troponin I: negative.
Chest X-ray: mild cardiomegaly.
Echocardiogram: mild aortic stenosis and mild mitral regurgitation. Left ventricular function mildly impaired (ejection fraction 46 per cent).

Questions

1 What does this ECG show?
2 What is the mechanism of this?
3 What are the likely causes?
4 What are the key issues in managing this patient?

2 Conduction between atria and ventricles has been interrupted.

3 Causes of third-degree atrioventricular block include idiopathic fibrosis of the atrioventricular junction and/or bundle branches. Other causes are acute myocardial infarction; aortic valve disease; cardiac surgery; infiltration by sarcoid, haemochromatosis, amyloid, tumour; inflammation due to endocarditis, rheumatic fever; Chagas' disease; Lyme disease; dystrophia myotonica.

4 The ventricular rate can be maintained with a temporary or permanent pacemaker. A physiological (DDDR) permanent pacemaker should restore the patient to normal daily activities.

ECG analysis

Rate	43 bpm
Rhythm	Sinus rhythm with third-degree atrioventricular block
QRS axis	Right axis deviation (+122°)
P waves	Normal
PR interval	Variable – there is no correlation between P waves and QRS complexes
QRS duration	Prolonged (122 ms)
T waves	Normal
QTc interval	Prolonged (510 ms)

Answers

1 This ECG shows third-degree atrioventricular block with a narrow QRS complex escape rhythm at 43 bpm. This is third-degree or **complete heart block**.

Commentary

● In third-degree atrioventricular block there is total disruption of the transmission of atrial impulses to the ventricles either at or below the atrioventricular node:

- when the block is within the atrioventricular node, subsidiary pacemakers arise, often within the bundle of His so that discharge is at a reliable and fairly fast rate and complexes are narrow.
- when there is infra-nodal block, subsidiary pacemakers arise in the bundle branches and so complexes are typically broad and the ventricular rate slow. Bundle pacemakers are less reliable and so Stokes–Adams attacks are more likely.

● A temporary pacemaker can be inserted via the subclavian, internal jugular, femoral or antecubital vein. In complete heart block due to acute inferior myocardial infarction, the left ventricle is usually spared, cardiac output is maintained and a temporary pacemaker is rarely necessary as normal conduction is usually restored within days. In complete heart block due to acute anterior infarction, infarction is more extensive and the combination of slow heart rate and left ventricular dysfunction results in poor cardiac output and a worse prognosis. A temporary pacemaker will maintain cardiac output to some extent but mortality remains high.

● Third-degree (complete) heart block should be distinguished from atrioventricular dissociation. In complete heart block the ventricular rate is lower than the atrial rate, as is the case here. In atrioventricular dissociation, the ventricular rate is the same as or higher than the atrial rate. Atrioventricular dissociation occurs when the sinoatrial node slows so much that a subsidiary pacemaker takes over, or when a subsidiary pacemaker speeds up and overtakes the sinoatrial node.

Further reading

Making Sense of the ECG: Conduction disturbances, p 58; Third-degree AV block, p 123; Pacemakers, p 222.

CASE 49

LOC 00000-0000   Speed: 25mm/sec   Limb: 20mm/mV   Chest: 20mm/mV

50~ 0.15-150 Hz

15725

Clinical scenario

Male, aged 40 years.

Presenting complaint
Hypertension.

History of presenting complaint
Patient noted to be hypertensive (152/94) during routine check-up. This ECG was performed as part of his cardiovascular assessment.

Past medical history
Recently diagnosed hypertension – not on medication.

Examination
Pulse: 64 bpm, regular.
Blood pressure: 152/94.
JVP: not elevated.
Heart sounds: normal.
Chest auscultation: unremarkable.
No peripheral oedema.

Investigations
FBC: Hb 15.3, WCC 6.1, platelets 409.
U&E: Na 141, K 4.3, urea 5.9, creatinine 83.
Chest X-ray: normal heart size, clear lung fields.

Questions

1 What does this ECG show?
2 What would you do next?

ECG analysis

Rate	64 bpm
Rhythm	Sinus rhythm
QRS axis	Normal (+32°)
P waves	Normal
PR interval	Normal (160 ms)
QRS duration	Normal (70 ms)
T waves	Normal
QTc interval	Normal (430 ms)

Additional comments

The voltage calibration setting is 20 mm/mV, double the 'standard' setting.

Answers

1 At first glance, this ECG might appear to meet a number of the diagnostic criteria for left ventricular hypertrophy (see Case 35). However, on closer inspection it can be seen that the voltage calibration has been set at 20 mm/mV, which is double the standard setting (10 mm/mV). Therefore all the waves/complexes on the ECG will be twice their 'usual' size. When this is taken into account, the ECG is in fact **normal**.

2 The ECG should be repeated at the standard calibration setting of 10 mm/mV (unless a different non-standard setting is required for a particular purpose).

Commentary

● ECGs are normally recorded at a standard calibration setting of 10 mm/mV. In other words, a voltage of 1 mV will cause a 10 mm deflection in the ECG tracing.

● The calibration setting is usually indicated on the ECG by an annotation (in this case 'Limb: 20 mm/mV Chest: 20 mm/mV' along the bottom of the ECG), and/or by a calibration marker (the upright 'box' at the far right of this recording, which shows what deflection is made by a voltage of 1 mV). It is good practice to check the calibration settings on every ECG you examine.

● Many ECG machines will allow the calibration of the limb leads and the chest leads to be set independently.

● For the vast majority of ECGs, a standard setting of 10 mm/mV is appropriate. For patients with very large QRS complexes (e.g. as seen in left ventricular hypertrophy), sometimes at the standard setting the QRS complexes on adjacent lines can overlap and make interpretation difficult. Under these circumstances, a calibration of 5 mm/mV will halve the size of the complexes and may make the ECG easier to interpret. The use of double the normal calibration (20 mm/mV) is very unusual.

Further reading
Making Sense of the ECG: How do I record an ECG? p 16; Incorrect calibration, p 219.

CASE 50

Speed: 25 mm/s   Limb: 10 mm/mV   Chest: 10 mm/mV

Clinical scenario

Male, aged 29 years.

Presenting complaint
Chest pain.

History of presenting complaint
Usually fit and well. Patient was at a party with friends
and had consumed quite a lot of alcohol – more than he
usually drank. Friends reported that he then developed
severe central chest pain which got progressively worse.
They were concerned so called for an ambulance.
Admitted to coronary care unit with a suspected acute
myocardial infarction.

Past medical history
Nil of note.
Heavy smoker.

Examination
Pulse: 48 bpm, some variation with respiration.
Blood pressure: 148/96.
JVP: not elevated.
Heart sounds: normal.
Chest auscultation: unremarkable.
No peripheral oedema.

Investigations
FBC: Hb 13.9, WCC 8.1, platelets 233.
U&E: Na 137, K 4.2, urea 5.3, creatinine 88.
Troponin I: negative.
Chest X-ray: normal heart size, clear lung fields.
Echocardiogram: normal valves. Left ventricular
function good (ejection fraction 67 per cent).

Questions

1 What does this ECG show?
2 What is the mechanism of this?
3 What are the likely causes?
4 What are the key issues in managing this patient?

ECG analysis

Rate	48 bpm
Rhythm	Sinus rhythm (with a degree of sinus arrhythmia)
QRS axis	Normal (+74°)
P waves	Normal
PR interval	Prolonged (232 ms)
QRS duration	Normal (114 ms)
T waves	Tall in V_2–V_4 ('hyperacute')
QTc interval	Normal (351 ms)

Additional comments
There is ST segment elevation in leads V_2–V_6.

Answers

1 ST segment elevation most marked in the anterior chest leads. If these changes resolve as the chest pain resolves, and there is no subsequent troponin rise, this is consistent with myocardial ischaemia due to **coronary artery vasospasm** ('Prinzmetal's angina').

2 Coronary artery vasospasm leads to a reduction in blood supply to myocardium supplied by the affected artery. ECG changes are not confined to the ST segment – hyperacute T waves, T wave inversion, or transient intraventricular conduction defects such as bundle branch or fascicular block may be evident.

3 While it can occur in normal arteries (it may be seen at coronary angiography on cannulating the right coronary artery, and cocaine is a potent stimulus), in 90 per cent of patients coronary artery vasospasm occurs at the site of atheroma. ST segment elevation may suggest an acute myocardial infarction, but with resolution of chest pain, the ST segments return to normal. It usually occurs at rest. Patients may also report symptoms of Raynaud's phenomenon. The patient in this case had been using cannabis prior to admission.

4 Treatment for Prinzmetal's (vasospastic) angina should include a calcium channel blocker and/or a nitrate.

Commentary

● Prinzmetal's or variant angina occurs almost exclusively at rest, is not usually brought on by exertion or emotion, and is associated with ST segment elevation which can occur in any lead – the risk of sudden death is increased if seen in both anterior and inferior leads. It may be associated with myocardial infarction and cardiac arrhythmias, including ventricular tachycardia, ventricular fibrillation and sudden death.

● Variant angina tends to affect younger patients than does chronic stable angina or unstable angina. Most will have few conventional risk factors other than heavy smoking. Illicit drug use with cannabis, a potent coronary vasoconstrictor and platelet activator, and cocaine, which causes alpha adrenergically mediated coronary constriction when 'snorted', should always be considered in a young person with severe chest pain, ST segment elevation and few risk factors.

● In patients prone to coronary artery spasm, coronary artery tone and responsiveness to constrictor stimuli are increased. A number of provocative tests have been developed, the most sensitive being ergonovine, an ergot alkaloid that stimulates alpha adrenergic and serotonin receptors which have a direct vasoconstrictive effect on vascular smooth muscle. It may be administered when coronary angiography has demonstrated normal coronary arteries. Hyperventilation is only slightly less sensitive than ergonovine. Most patients have underlying coronary disease and spasm tends to occur close to existing coronary lesions.

● Treatment is based on relieving the coronary spasm:
  ● calcium channel blockers
  ● nitrates.

  Beta blockers may *worsen* coronary spasm and should be avoided.

Further reading
Making Sense of the ECG: Prinzmetal's (vasospastic) angina, p 170.

CASE 51

Speed: 25 mm/s   Limb: 10 mm/mV   Chest: 10 mm/mV

Clinical scenario

Male, aged 55 years.

Presenting complaint

Syncopal episode while walking uphill.

History of presenting complaint

Three-month history of gradually worsening breathlessness and dizziness on exertion, culminating in a brief syncopal episode while walking uphill. An ambulance was called and the patient was brought to the hospital where this ECG was recorded.

Past medical history

Nil.

Examination

Patient comfortable at rest. Alert and oriented.
Pulse: 96 bpm, regular, slow rising.

Blood pressure: 108/86.
JVP: not elevated.
Precordium: left parasternal heave.
Heart sounds: loud (4/6) ejection systolic murmur heard in the aortic area, radiating to both carotid arteries.
Chest auscultation: unremarkable.
No peripheral oedema.

Investigations

FBC: Hb 13.8, WCC 7.1, platelets 388.
U&E: Na 141, K 4.4, urea 6.8, creatinine 112.
Chest X-ray: normal heart size, clear lung fields.

Questions

1 What does the ECG show?
2 What investigation would help to confirm this?
3 What can cause these appearances? What is the likely cause here?
4 What are the treatment options?

ECG analysis

Rate	96 bpm
Rhythm	Sinus rhythm
QRS axis	Normal ($+11°$)
P waves	Normal
PR interval	Normal (160 ms)
QRS duration	Normal (80 ms)
T waves	Inverted in leads I, aVL, V_4–V_6, and also in lead II
QTc interval	Prolonged (500 ms)

Additional comments

There are very deep S waves (up to 48 mm) in leads V_2–V_3 and very tall R waves (up to 44 mm) in leads V_5–V_6.

Answers

1 This ECG shows very deep S waves (up to 48 mm) in leads V_2–V_3 and very tall R waves (up to 44 mm) in leads V_5–V_6, together with inverted T waves in leads I, aVL, V_4–V_6 (and also in lead II). These appearances are indicative of left ventricular hypertrophy with 'strain'.

2 An echocardiogram (or cardiac magnetic resonance scan) would allow direct visualization of the left ventricle, assessment of the extent of left ventricular hypertrophy, assessment of left ventricular systolic (and diastolic) function, and also assessment of the structure and function of the aortic valve.

3 Left ventricular hypertrophy can result from:
- hypertension
- aortic stenosis
- coarctation of the aorta
- hypertrophic cardiomyopathy.

The clinical findings indicate that aortic stenosis is the most likely cause of left ventricular hypertrophy in this case.

4 Where left ventricular hypertrophy is secondary to pressure overload of the left ventricle, the appropriate treatment is that of the underlying cause. In the case of aortic stenosis, the aortic valve must be assessed by echocardiography (or cardiac magnetic resonance scanning) and, if severe symptomatic aortic stenosis is confirmed, plans should be made for surgical aortic valve replacement.

Commentary

● The diagnostic ECG criteria for left ventricular hypertrophy were discussed earlier in Case 35. The ECG in the present case meets several of these diagnostic criteria:

● In the chest leads:
  – R wave of 25 mm or more in the left chest leads
  – S wave of 25 mm or more in the right chest leads
  – Sum of S wave in lead V_1 and R wave in lead V_5 or V_6 greater than 35 mm (Sokolow–Lyon criteria)

● Sum of tallest R wave and deepest S wave in the chest leads greater than 45 mm.

● The Cornell criteria are met:
  – The Cornell criteria involve measuring S wave in lead V_3 and the R wave in lead aVL. Left ventricular hypertrophy is indicated by a sum of >28 mm in men and >20 mm in women.

● The ECG also meets the Romhilt–Estes criteria for left ventricular hypertrophy, scoring 6 points:
  – S wave in right chest leads of 25 mm or more, and also R wave in left chest leads of 25 mm or more (3 points)

  – ST segment and T wave changes ('typical strain') in a patient not taking digitalis (3 points).

● The presence of ST segment depression and/or T wave inversion in the context of left ventricular hypertrophy are taken to indicate left ventricular 'strain'. However, it is important to assess the clinical context – ST/T wave changes, particularly if dynamic, associated with symptoms of chest pain may instead indicate myocardial ischaemia.

● The risk of myocardial infarction and stroke in patients with left ventricular hypertrophy with a strain pattern is approximately double that of patients who have left ventricular hypertrophy without strain.

Further reading

Making Sense of the ECG: Left ventricular hypertrophy, p 136; Ventricular hypertrophy with 'strain', p 182.

CASE 52

Speed: 25 mm/s   Limb: 10 mm/mV   Chest: 10 mm/mV

Clinical scenario

Male, aged 64 years.

Presenting complaint

Severe chest pain ('tight band' around chest), associated with breathlessness. Felt dizzy and fainted.

History of presenting complaint

Digging in garden all day. Ignored chest pain earlier in day.

Past medical history

High blood pressure for several years.

Was a heavy smoker until 4 weeks ago.

Strong family history of coronary artery disease.

Examination

Pulse: 90 bpm, regular.

Blood pressure: 92/70.

JVP: elevated by 3 cm.

Heart sounds: normal.

Chest auscultation: unremarkable.

Mild peripheral oedema.

Investigations

FBC: Hb 14.4, WCC 11.2, platelets 332.

U&E: Na 143, K 4.6, urea 5.4, creatinine 108.

Troponin I: elevated at 6.6 (after 12 h).

Chest X-ray: normal heart size, clear lung fields.

Echocardiogram: normal valve function. Inferior hypokinesia of left ventricle (ejection fraction 48 per cent); right ventricle – impaired function.

Questions

1 What sort of ECG recording is this?
2 What does this ECG show?
3 What treatment would be appropriate in this patient?

ECG analysis

Rate	90 bpm
Rhythm	Sinus rhythm
QRS axis	Normal (+20°)
P waves	Normal
PR interval	Normal (160 ms)
QRS duration	Normal (110 ms)
T waves	Normal
QTc interval	Prolonged (490 ms)

Additional comments

There is inferior ST segment elevation with reciprocal lateral ST segment depression. The right-sided chest leads show ST segment elevation in leads V$_3$R–V$_6$R.

Answers

1 This is an ECG showing the usual limb leads but **right-sided chest leads** (V$_1$R–V$_6$R). An ECG with right-sided chest leads should be performed in all patients presenting with an acute inferior myocardial infarction, to look for evidence of right ventricular involvement (as shown by ST segment elevation in lead V$_4$R).

2 The ECG shows an **acute inferior STEMI** (ST segment elevation in leads II, III, aVF) with reciprocal ST segment depression laterally (leads I and aVL). There is ST segment elevation in leads V$_3$R–V$_6$R. The presence of ST segment elevation in lead V$_4$R is indicative of **right ventricular involvement.**

3 Aspirin 300 mg orally (then 75 mg once daily), clopidogrel 300 mg orally (then 75 mg once daily for one month), glyceryl trinitrate sublingually, pain relief (diamorphine, plus an anti-emetic), oxygen. Prompt restoration of myocardial blood flow is required, either through primary percutaneous coronary intervention (PCI) or, if primary PCI is not available, thrombolysis. In right ventricular infarction, hypotension may be the result of reduced left ventricular filling pressures (as a result of right ventricular impairment) and so careful fluid management is essential.

Commentary

● The prognosis in inferior myocardial infarction is generally very good. However, when the infarction involves the right ventricle (about 50 per cent of cases), the risk of severe complications is increased almost sixfold:

- death, ventricular fibrillation, re-infarction.
- risk of right-sided heart failure (elevated JVP, peripheral oedema, low output state but with no evidence of pulmonary oedema).

● In inferior myocardial infarction with right ventricular involvement, hypotension is usually due to poor right ventricular contractility secondary to the right ventricular infarction. Volume expansion with aliquots of 250 mL of normal saline intravenously, repeated as necessary, may be effective in maintaining right ventricular output and thus left ventricular filling pressure. Failure to respond warrants consideration of right- and left-sided filling pressure monitoring using a Swan–Ganz catheter – high right-sided pressures and a low pulmonary capillary wedge (= left atrial) pressure confirms right ventricular infarction. It is essential to avoid vasodilator drugs which may reduce the right ventricular output even further.

Further reading

Making Sense of the ECG: Are the ST segments elevated? p 159; Why is right ventricular infarction important? p 168. Chockalingam A, Gnanavelu G, Subramaniam, T. Right ventricular myocardial infarction: presentation and acute outcomes. *Angiology* 2005; **56**: 371–6.

CASE 53

Clinical scenario

Male, aged 22 years.

Presenting complaint
Fatigue.

History of presenting complaint
Longstanding history of fatigue.
No other associated symptoms.

Past medical history
Childhood asthma – no longer uses inhalers.

Examination
Pulse: 58 bpm, regular.
Blood pressure: 124/76.
JVP: not elevated.
Heart sounds: normal.
Chest auscultation: unremarkable.
No peripheral oedema.

Investigations
FBC: Hb 15.5, WCC 5.2, platelets 389.
U&E: Na 143, K 4.9, urea 3.6, creatinine 67.
Thyroid function: normal.

Questions

1 What does this ECG show?
2 What would you do next?
3 What is the cause of this patient's fatigue?

ECG analysis

Rate	58 bpm
Rhythm	Sinus rhythm (slight bradycardia)
QRS axis	Unable to assess (single lead)
P waves	Present
PR interval	Normal (160 ms)
QRS duration	Normal (80 ms)
T waves	Normal
QTc interval	Normal (413 ms)

Additional comments
The paper speed is set at 50 mm/s, double the normal recording speed.

Answers

1 This ECG shows normal sinus rhythm with a heart rate of 58 bpm (slight bradycardia). At first glance, the rate looks like it might be slower than that (29 bpm), but that is because the recording has been made a double the normal paper speed (50 mm/s) rather than the standard 25 mm/s). The paper speed is shown at the lower left corner of the rhythm strip.

2 The ECG should be repeated at the standard paper setting of 25 mm/s.

3 This ECG rhythm strip does not reveal an explanation for this patient's fatigue – his heart rate is virtually normal at 58 bpm. Further clinical assessment is required to identify the cause of his fatigue.

Commentary

● The standard ECG paper speed in the UK and the USA is 25 mm/s, which makes each small square equivalent to 0.04 s and each large square equivalent to 0.2 s. By counting large and/or small squares, you can calculate such parameters as heart rate and PR and QT intervals.

● If a 'non-standard' paper speed is used, the 'time value' of small and large squares need to be adjusted accordingly. At 50 mm/s, the small squares will equal 0.02 s and the large squares 0.1 s. All measurements and calculations must take the new speed setting into account.

● A speed setting of 50 mm/s is sometimes used to make measurements easier (by doubling the width of

every wave, some features can be seen and/or measured more easily). A paper speed of 50 mm/s is used as the standard setting in some parts of Europe, rather than 25 mm/s.

● All ECGs should be annotated with the paper speed that was used for the recording. If a non-standard paper speed was used, this should be highlighted clearly to avoid misinterpretation.

● When an ECG has been recorded using a non-standard paper speed in error, it should be repeated using the appropriate paper speed.

Further reading

Making Sense of the ECG: How do I record an ECG? p 16; Incorrect paper speed, p 220.

CASE 54

Speed: 25 mm/s   Limb: 10 mm/mV   Chest: 10 mm/mV

Clinical scenario

Male, aged 22 years.

Presenting complaint
Admitted with lower respiratory tract infection.

History of presenting complaint
Cough, productive of blood-stained sputum; fever;
tachycardia

Past medical history
Nil of note.

Examination
Pulse: 76 bpm, irregularly irregular.
Blood pressure: 134/76.

JVP: not elevated.
Heart sounds: quiet; heard best on right side of chest.
Chest auscultation: bronchial breathing right lower
lobe.
No peripheral oedema.

Investigations
FBC: Hb 15.6, WCC 13.5, platelets 224.
U&E: Na 139, K 3.9, urea 4.4, creatinine 86.
Chest X-ray: dextrocardia; consolidation right lower
lobe.
Echocardiogram: dextrocardia. Normal valves. Left
ventricular function normal (ejection fraction 67
per cent).

Questions

1 What abnormalities does this ECG show?
2 What are the likely causes?
3 What are the key issues in managing this patient?

ECG analysis

Rate	76 bpm
Rhythm	Atrial fibrillation
QRS axis	Extreme right axis deviation (+124°)
P waves	Absent (atrial fibrillation)
PR interval	N/A
QRS duration	Normal (112 ms)
T waves	Normal
QTc interval	Normal (446 ms)

Additional comments
There is a decrease in QRS complex size from lead V_1 to lead V_6.

Answers

1 The rhythm is atrial fibrillation. Leads I and aVL are negative and leads II, III and aVR are positive – this is extreme right axis deviation. The R waves are generally small across the chest leads, and *decrease* in size from V_1 to V_6 (normally, the R waves are small in V_1, equipolar at V_3 or V_4 and largest at V_6).

2 This is **dextrocardia**. Dextrocardia is a naturally occurring anomaly, seen in 1:10000 people. The ECG 'abnormalities' occur because the recording reflects the heart's abnormal position in the thorax. The ECG will 'normalize' if the chest leads are reversed so that lead V_1 is recorded from the *left* sternal edge and V_6 from the *right* axilla. The patient's atrial fibrillation is likely to have been triggered by the lower respiratory tract infection, but a careful review for other possible causes should always be undertaken.

3 The ECG 'abnormalities' seen in dextrocardia must not be considered pathological – the heart is usually structurally normal. It is important that the finding of dextrocardia be recorded prominently in a patient's notes to prevent mishaps, especially during emergency surgery. The patient's atrial fibrillation should be managed in the same way as any other patient with atrial fibrillation (see Case 6).

Commentary

● The term *situs* describes the position of the cardiac atria and viscera, cardiac situs being determined by atrial location, so:
  ● situs solitus – is the normal orientation of viscera and a left-sided heart
  ● situs inversus – is reversal of all the major structures in the thorax and abdomen
  ● situs ambiguous – the orientation of heart and viscera conform to neither situs solitus nor inversus (any structure with a right-left asymmetry can be normal, completely reversed or neither).

● In situs inversus with levocardia, the apex of the heart points to the left; with dextrocardia, it points to the right. Dextrocardia on its own is known as situs solitus with dextrocardia.

● Other congenital cardiovascular abnormalities can be associated with dextrocardia, such as single ventricle, atrial or ventricular septal defects, anomalous pulmonary venous return, and transposition of the great arteries. When dextrocardia occurs with just the heart incorrectly positioned, functionally significant complex cardiac abnormalities are more likely.

● Situs inversus totalis may be associated with ciliary dysfunction (Kartagener's syndrome) in which patients experience repeated sinus and respiratory infections resulting in bronchiectasis, chronic sinusitis and nasal polyposis. Life expectancy is normal if bronchiectasis is adequately treated.

Further reading
Making Sense of the ECG: Dextrocardia, p 142.

CASE 55

Speed: 25 mm/s   Limb: 10 mm/mV   Chest: 10 mm/mV

Figure adapted with permission from the BMJ Publishing Group (*Heart* 2003; **89**: 1363–72).

Clinical scenario

Female, aged 47 years.

Presenting complaint
Post-cardiac arrest (ventricular fibrillation).

History of presenting complaint
Patient presented with a ventricular fibrillation cardiac arrest. This ECG was recorded immediately after successful resuscitation.

Past medical history
Treated with thioridazine 20 mg daily (an antipsychotic drug used in the treatment of schizophrenia and psychosis).

Examination
Post-cardiac arrest.
Pulse: 84 bpm, regular.
Blood pressure: 134/82.
JVP: not elevated.
Heart sounds: normal.
Chest auscultation: unremarkable.
No peripheral oedema.

Investigations
FBC: Hb 12.9, WCC 9.0, platelets 316.
U&E: Na 139, K 4.6, urea 5.4, creatinine 95.
Chest X-ray: normal heart size, clear lung fields.
Echocardiogram: normal.

Questions

1 What does this ECG show?
2 What can cause this abnormality?
3 What treatment is appropriate?

ECG analysis

Rate	84 bpm
Rhythm	Sinus rhythm
QRS axis	Normal (+29°)
P waves	Normal
PR interval	Normal (160 ms)
QRS duration	Normal (80 ms)
T waves	Normal
QTc interval	Prolonged (619 ms)

Answers

1 This ECG shows a very prolonged QTc interval of 619 ms.
2 Causes of QTc prolongation include:
  • congential long QT syndromes
  • drug effects (see Commentary)
  • hypokalaemia, hypocalcaemia, hypomagnesaemia
  • acute myocarditis.

QTc prolongation can sometimes also be seen in cases of acute myocardial infarction, cerebral injury, hypertrophic cardiomyopathy and hypothermia.

3 The QTc returned to normal (399 ms) three days after withdrawal of thioridazine.

Commentary

● The normal QT interval varies with heart rate, becoming shorter at faster rates. Measurements of the QT interval therefore need to be correct for heart rate. The most common method for calculating the corrected QT interval (QTc) is Bazett's formula, dividing the measured QT interval by the square root of the RR interval (all measurements in seconds). A normal QTc interval is 350–440 ms, although QT intervals tend to be a little longer in women than in men, and so some authorities quote a normal QTc of up to 440 ms in men and 450 ms (and sometimes up to 460 ms) in women. Long QT intervals are associated with a risk of polymorphic ventricular tachycardia (torsades de pointes), which is discussed in Case 61.

● Long QT intervals can be congenital or acquired. A number of hereditary syndromes are now grouped together as long QT syndrome (LQTS), in which genetic abnormalities of the potassium or sodium channels leads to prolonged ventricular repolarization and hence prolongation of the QT interval. The most common long QT syndromes are LQT1 and LQT2 (potassium channel abnormalities) and LQT3 (sodium channel abnormality). This classification includes the hereditary Romano–Ward syndrome and the Jervell and Lange–Nielsen syndrome.

● Acquired causes include drug-induced QT prolongation, which is caused by the drug effect on the heart's I_{Kr} potassium channel. A large number of drugs can prolong the QT interval, including certain anti-arrhythmic drugs, antipsychotics, tricyclic antidepressants, non-sedating antihistamines, antimicrobials and antimalarials.

Further reading

Making Sense of the ECG: Torsades de pointes (polymorphic VT), p 56; Is the QTc interval longer than 0.44s? p 207.
Yap YG, Camm AJ. Drug induced QT prolongation and torsades de pointes. *Heart* 2003; **89**: 1363–72.

CASE 56

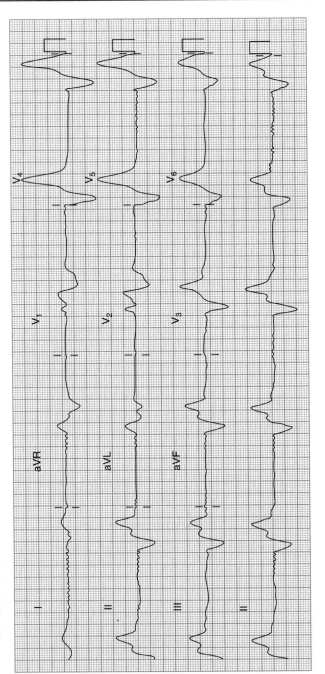

Clinical scenario

Male, aged 72 years.

Presenting complaint

Severe central chest pain.

History of presenting complaint

Patient currently an inpatient on the coronary care unit.
He had an acute myocardial infarction 36 h previously.

Past medical history

Hypertension.
Type 2 diabetes mellitus.

Examination

Pulse: 36 bpm, regular.
Blood pressure: 124/88.
JVP: not elevated.

Heart sounds: normal.
Chest auscultation: unremarkable.
No peripheral oedema.

Investigations

FBC: Hb 12.4, WCC 9.6, platelets 256.
U&E: Na 139, K 4.1, urea 4.3, creatinine 128.
Troponin I: elevated at 7.8 (after 12 h).
Chest X-ray: mild cardiomegaly, early pulmonary congestion.
Echocardiogram: left ventricular function mildly impaired (ejection fraction 47 per cent).

Questions

1 What does this ECG show?
2 What is the mechanism of this?
3 What are the likely causes?
4 What are the key issues in managing this patient?

ECG analysis

Rate	36 bpm
Rhythm	Regular
QRS axis	Left axis deviation (−90°)
P waves	Absent
PR interval	N/A
QRS duration	Prolonged (220 ms)
T waves	Normal
QTc interval	Prolonged (464 ms)

Answers

1 The QRS complexes are wide and appear in a regular rhythm. This is a 'slow' form of monomorphic ventricular tachycardia', sometimes called "idioventricular rhythm' or 'accelerated idioventricular rhythm'.

2 Idioventricular rhythm is caused by enhanced automaticity of His–Purkinje fibres or myocardium, appearing under specific metabolic conditions such as acute myocardial ischaemia (the most common), hypoxaemia, hypokalaemia or digoxin toxicity. These conditions increase the rate of impulse generation in pacemaker tissues usually subordinate to the sinus node, which escape from sinus control.

3 It is usually seen in the first two days after an acute myocardial infarction. When seen after thrombolysis, it is usually accepted as a marker of successful coronary reperfusion.

4 The rhythm abnormality is benign and treatment is necessary only if there is haemodynamic compromise.

Commentary

● Sometimes called 'slow VT', idioventricular rhythm:
  • is a benign form of ventricular tachycardia
  • it is equally common in inferior and anterior myocardial infarction
  • often occurs as an escape rhythm during slowing of the sinus rate
  • usually has a rate of 60–120 bpm with a QRS complex duration >120 ms (in the case presented here, the rate is significantly lower).

● Rarely, the ventricular rate may increase, causing ventricular tachycardia or ventricular fibrillation. Treatment then involves increasing the sinus rate with atropine or atrial pacing.

Further reading
Making Sense of the ECG: Accelerated idioventricular rhythm, p. 56.

CASE 57

Speed: 25 mm/sec   Limb: 10 mm/mV   Chest: 10 mm/mV

Clinical scenario

Female, aged 77 years.

Presenting complaint
Haematemesis and melaena.

History of presenting complaint
Patient had been taking non-steroidal anti-inflammatory drugs for the past 4 weeks to obtain pain relief from her osteoarthritis. She presented with haematemesis, having vomited approximately 500 mL of fresh blood, and subsequently developed melaena.

Past medical history
Osteoarthritis.
Ischaemic heart disease.

Examination
Clammy, pale.
Pulse: 120 bpm, regular.
Blood pressure: 86/46.
JVP: not seen.
Heart sounds: normal.
Chest auscultation: unremarkable.
No peripheral oedema.

Investigations
FBC: Hb 6.8, WCC 13.2, platelets 309.
U&E: Na 137, K 4.1, urea 16.7, creatinine 93.
Chest X-ray: normal heart size, clear lung fields.
Gastroscopy: large, actively bleeding duodenal ulcer.

Questions

1 What does this ECG show?
2 What would you do about the heart rate?

ECG analysis

Rate	120 bpm
Rhythm	Sinus tachycardia
QRS axis	Normal (+48°)
P waves	Present
PR interval	Normal (120 ms)
QRS duration	Broad (130 ms)
T waves	Normal
QTc interval	Normal (450 ms)

Additional comments

The QRS complexes have a left bundle branch block morphology.

Answers

1 This ECG shows a tachycardia (heart rate 120 bpm) with broad QRS complexes (QRS duration 130 ms). The QRS complexes have a left bundle branch block (LBBB) morphology. On careful inspection, P waves can be seen before the QRS complexes – the P waves are most easily seen in lead V$_1$. This broad-complex tachycardia is therefore sinus tachycardia with aberrant conduction (LBBB).

2 This patient's sinus tachycardia is appropriate to her haemodynamic state – she has lost blood and is hypotensive, and has therefore developed a sinus tachycardia to help maintain cardiac output. Trying to slow down the tachycardia in these circumstances would be dangerous, causing haemodynamic decompensation. The management of sinus tachycardia therefore depends critically on the identification and, where possible, treatment of the underlying cause. The appropriate action here would be to correct the hypovolaemia and to prevent any further blood loss.

Commentary

● Broad-complex tachycardia (QRS complex duration >120 ms) can result from:

- ventricular tachycardia (VT)
- supraventricular tachycardia (SVT) with aberrant conduction
- ventricular pacing.

● If a patient has a pre-existing bundle branch block in normal sinus rhythm, that bundle branch block will also remain present during episodes of SVT. However, some patients may have normal QRS complexes while in normal sinus rhythm, but develop a bundle branch block only during episodes of tachycardia ('functional' bundle branch block). In such cases, the development of functional right bundle branch block (RBBB) is more common than functional left bundle branch block (LBBB). Sudden changes in RR interval (as seen, for example, in atrial fibrillation) are particularly likely to cause functional bundle branch block – this is referred to as the Ashman phenomenon.

● Supraventricular tachycardia with aberrant conduction also includes SVT occurring with ventricular pre-excitation, for example antidromic atrioventricular re-entry tachycardia or atrial fibrillation with pre-excitation, both of which can occur in Wolff–Parkinson–White syndrome (see Case 59).

● Distinguishing between VT and SVT with aberrant conduction can be challenging. If the QRS morphology has a typical RBBB or LBBB, then it is likely to be SVT with aberrant conduction. However, this is certainly not diagnostic as some forms of VT can resemble LBBB or RBBB very closely. If the QRS complexes are very broad (RBBB morphology with QRS duration >140 ms, LBBB morphology with QRS duration >160 ms), then VT is more likely. An extreme QRS axis (between −90° and −180°) also points towards VT, as do concordant negative QRS complexes in the chest leads. One of the most valuable criteria for diagnosing VT is the presence of independent atrial activity (see Commentary, Case 58).

● Broad-complex tachycardia should always be managed as VT until proven otherwise.

Further reading

Making Sense of the ECG: Sinus tachycardia, p 32; How do I distinguish between VT and SVT? p 74; Bundle branch block, p 147.

Eckardt L, Breithardt G, Kirchhof, P. Approach to wide complex tachycardias in patients without structural heart disease. *Heart* 2006; **92**: 704–11.

CASE 58

Clinical scenario

Male, aged 76 years.

Presenting complaint

Chest pain and breathlessness.

History of presenting complaint

Patient was woken from sleep by severe chest pain and breathlessness.

Past medical history

Myocardial infarction 12 months previously. Treated with thrombolysis. Occasional chest pain on exertion at intervals since. Had reduced activities to avoid chest pain.

Examination

Pulse: 152 bpm, regular.
Blood pressure: 108/72.

JVP: not elevated.
Heart sounds: normal.
Chest auscultation: unremarkable.
No peripheral oedema.

Investigations

FBC: Hb 12.8, WCC 6.3, platelets 267.
U&E: Na 135, K 3.2, urea 8.2, creatinine 138.
Thyroid function: normal.
Troponin I: negative.
Chest X-ray: marked cardiomegaly with signs of pulmonary congestion.
Echocardiogram: moderate mitral regurgitation into moderately dilated left atrium. Left ventricular function severely impaired (ejection fraction 25 per cent).

Questions

1 What does this ECG show?
2 What are the key issues in managing this patient?

ECG analysis

Rate	152 bpm
Rhythm	Ventricular tachycardia
QRS axis	+93°
P waves	Not seen
PR interval	N/A
QRS duration	Prolonged (164 ms)
T waves	Not clearly seen
QTc interval	T waves not clearly seen

Answers

1 This ECG shows a broad-complex tachycardia. There is positive concordance of the anterior chest leads (the QRS complexes in the anterior leads are all positive). This is **ventricular tachycardia (VT)**.

2 *Acute management*
• Cardiopulmonary resuscitation – if the patient is haemodynamically compromised, the appropriate protocols should be followed including electrical cardioversion (otherwise intravenous amiodarone or lidocaine).
• Manage the underlying cause (e.g. acute coronary syndrome) as appropriate.

3 *Long term management*
• Aim to prevent recurrence and reduce the risk of sudden death
• Asymptomatic non-sustained VT with low risk (preserved LV function) – no treatment needed.
• Symptomatic non-sustained VT – Class IC/II/III anti-arrhythmic drugs.
• Post-MI non-sustained VT with poor LV function (LVEF 35–40 per cent): undertake electrophysiological studies – if inducible VT not suppressed by drugs, there is a mortality benefit of using an implantable cardioverter-fibrillator (ICD).
• Ischaemic cardiomyopathy (previous MI) with LVEF <30 per cent: ICD is superior to medical treatment.
• Post-cardiac arrest/sustained VT with LVEF <35 per cent: ICD. If unacceptable to patient, use amiodarone empirically.
• Recurrent shocks post-ICD: amiodarone to slow rate or allow overdrive pacing. Alternatives: sotalol, procain-amide, mexiletine. Combinations of drugs may be necessary.
• Post-cardiac arrest/sustained VT with LVEF >35 per cent: amiodarone.
• Post-infarct VT well-tolerated and with good left ventricular function: electrophysiological studies and ablation, or amiodarone or sotalol.

- Class II/III heart failure with sustained VT without syncope or cardiac arrest – ICD recommended.
- The treatment of choice in life-threatening VT is the implantable defibrillator.

Commentary

- It can be difficult to differentiate VT and supraventricular tachycardia with aberrant conduction (if in doubt, always manage as VT until proven otherwise).
- ECG findings favouring ventricular tachycardia:
  - a broad complex tachycardia in a patient with a history of coronary disease (especially myocardial infarction)
  - QRS duration in tachycardia – the wider the QRS, the more likely the rhythm is to be VT (VT is the most common cause of tachycardia with a broad QRS)
  - normal QRS duration in sinus rhythm but >140 ms during tachycardia
  - marked change in axis (whether to the left or right), compared with ECG in sinus rhythm
  - concordance – the QRS complexes in the chest leads are all positive or negative.

- Evidence of independent atrial activity is strongly supportive of a diagnosis of VT:
  - atrioventricular dissociation – P waves occurring with no relation to the QRS complexes
  - capture beats – an atrial impulse manages to 'capture' the ventricles for one beat, causing a normal QRS complex, which may be preceded by a P wave
  - fusion beats – these appear when the ventricles are activated by an atrial impulse and a ventricular impulse simultaneously.

Further reading

Making Sense of the ECG: Ventricular tachycardia, p 53; How do I distinguish between VT and SVT? p 74.

National Institute for Health and Clinical Excellence. *Implantable cardioverter defibrillators (ICDs) for the treatment of arrhythmias (review of TA11)*. Technology appraisal 95. London: NICE, 2006. Available at: www.nice.org.uk/ta95.

CASE 59

Figure adapted with permission from the BMJ Publishing Group (*Heart* 2006; **92**: 704–11).

Clinical scenario

Male, aged 28 years.

Presenting complaint

Palpitations, breathlessness and dizziness.

History of presenting complaint

This patient with known Wolff–Parkinson–White syndrome presented with a 1-h episode of rapid regular palpitation associated with dizziness and breathlessness.

Past medical history

Wolff–Parkinson–White syndrome.

Examination

Pulse: 240 bpm, regular.
Blood pressure: 108/64.
Heart sounds: difficult to discern individual heart sounds in view of tachycardia.
Chest auscultation: unremarkable.
No peripheral oedema.

Investigations

FBC: Hb 15.2, WCC 7.4, platelets 413.
U&E: Na 142, K 4.9, urea 4.2, creatinine 66.
Thyroid function: normal.

Questions

1 What rhythm is shown on this ECG?
2 Is this related to the patient's Wolff–Parkinson–White syndrome?
3 What treatment would be appropriate?

ECG analysis

Rate	240 bpm
Rhythm	Atrioventricular re-entry tachycardia (antidromic)
QRS axis	Right axis deviation (+135°)
P waves	Present as a deflection after the QRS complexes
PR interval	Not applicable
QRS duration	Broad complexes (192 ms)
T waves	Difficult to discern morphology in view of tachycardia
QTc interval	–

Answers

1 This ECG shows a regular broad-complex tachycardia with a heart rate of 240 bpm. The differential diagnosis includes antidromic atrioventricular re-entry tachycardia (AVRT) or ventricular tachycardia (VT). In this case, the patient proved to have antidromic AVRT, but it is entirely reasonable to regard any broad-complex tachycardia as VT until proven otherwise.

2 Yes – antidromic AVRT occurs when patients with Wolff–Parkinson–White syndrome develop a re-entry circuit which travels down the accessory pathway and back up the atrioventricular node. Most cases of AVRT in Wolff–Parkinson–White syndrome are orthodromic (see Commentary) but some cases are antidromic.

3 Antidromic AVRT can be treated in the same way as orthodromic AVRT, breaking the re-entry circuit by temporarily blocking the atrioventricular node (e.g. adenosine, carotid sinus massage, Valsalva manoeuvre). If the patient is haemodynamically compromised, or if VT is suspected, the arrhythmia can also be terminated with a synchronized DC shock.

CASE 60

Clinical scenario

Female, aged 36 years.

Presenting complaint
Breathlessness, intermittent chest pain and palpitations.

History of presenting complaint
Been slowing down at lot recently; had to abandon walking holiday in Scotland as very breathless on attempting to walk up hills.

Past medical history
Non-smoker.
No family history of cardiovascular disease but her sister is undergoing investigations for similar problems.

Examination
Pulse: 84 bpm, regular.
Blood pressure: 136/86.
JVP: not elevated.
Heart sounds: soft ejection systolic murmur in aortic area and lower left sternal edge.
Chest auscultation: unremarkable.
No peripheral oedema.

Investigations
FBC: Hb 12.9, WCC 7.8, platelets 259
U&E: Na 137, K 4.2, urea 5.3, creatinine 88.
Troponin I: negative.
Chest X-ray: mild cardiomegaly.

Questions

1 What does this ECG show?
2 What is the mechanism of this?
3 What are the likely causes?
4 What are the key issues in managing this patient?

ECG analysis

Rate	84 bpm
Rhythm	Sinus rhythm
QRS axis	Normal (−15°)
P waves	Normal
PR interval	Normal (198 ms)
QRS duration	Normal (100 ms)
T waves	Inverted I, aVL, V$_6$
QTc interval	Normal (450 ms)

Additional comments
There are deep Q waves in the anterior leads.

Answers

1 The deep anterior Q waves are suggestive of septal hypertrophy. Echocardiography confirmed that the patient had severe asymmetrical hypertrophy of the interventricular septum with obstruction to the left ventricular outflow tract – this is hypertrophic obstructive cardiomyopathy (HOCM).

2 ECG changes are due to thickened septal muscle – the most common variety of HOCM. If this is in the outflow tract, the Venturi effect of increased blood flow velocity during systole causes systolic anterior motion of mitral valve (and mitral regurgitation).

3 In 70 per cent, there is a genetic mutation in the gene coding for beta myosin, alpha-tropomyosin and troponin T. Inheritance is autosomal dominant, though 50 per cent of cases are sporadic.

4 An accurate diagnosis is important to establish whether there is obstruction to outflow from the left ventricle – the obstructive variety of cardiomyopathy carries a worse prognosis than non-obstructive. Investigate and monitor for rhythm abnormalities and treat with anti-arrhythmic drugs as appropriate – high risk patients may benefit from an implantable cardioverter defibrillator (ICD). Beta blockers or verapamil will reduce gradient across the outflow tract and control angina. In patients with more severe symptoms – reduce outflow tract obstruction by septal myomectomy either surgically or by alcohol ablation. Dual chamber pacing may improve symptoms and increase exercise tolerance. Screening of first-degree relatives is important.

Commentary

● Hypertrophic cardiomyopathy is a heterogeneous disease of the sarcomere with at least 150 different mutations in 10 different sarcomeric proteins. Certain mutations may delay penetrance so that the disease presents late (>60 years). Molecular genetic studies will become more widely available in future to assist diagnosis.

● The ECG may be normal, may show a mild degree of hypertrophy, or show left ventricular hypertrophy and 'strain', or sharply negative T waves in precordial leads V_1–V_3, deep Q waves, atrial fibrillation, ventricular ectopics or ventricular tachycardia. ECG changes are often evident before echocardiographic features, especially in the young.

● Characteristic features to look for on echocardiography – asymmetrical left ventricular hypertrophy, small left ventricular cavity, systolic anterior motion of the mitral valve, mitral regurgitation, and mid-systolic closure of the aortic valve.

● Magnetic resonance imaging may be required for definitive diagnosis.

● On identifying the index case, arrange echocardiography of first-degree relatives.

● Factors associated with a poor prognosis:

- young age
- family history of HOCM and sudden death
- sustained ventricular tachycardia
- presentation with syncope.

Further reading

Making Sense of the ECG: Left ventricular hypertrophy, p 136.

Wigle ED. Cardiomyopathy. The diagnosis of hypertrophic cardiomyopathy. *Heart* 2001; **86**: 709–14.

CASE 61

Speed: 25 mm/s   Limb: 10 mm/mV   Chest: 10 mm/mV

Clinical scenario

Female, aged 63 years.

Presenting complaint

Syncope.

History of presenting complaint

Patient admitted to hospital complaining of fatigue and muscle weakness after a week's history of diarrhoea and vomiting. She had a syncopal event shortly after admission and ECG monitoring was commenced. Shortly afterwards the patient had another syncopal episode and this ECG was recorded.

Past medical history

Alcoholic cirrhosis of the liver.

Examination

Clinical features of alcoholic liver disease with ascites.
Pulse: too fast to record manually.
Blood pressure: 96/54.
JVP: elevated by 6 cm.
Heart sounds: gallop rhythm.
Chest auscultation: bilateral pleural effusions.
Moderate peripheral oedema.

Investigations

FBC: Hb 10.8, WCC 18.1, platelets 124.
U&E: Na 127, K 2.3, urea 4.9, creatinine 85.
Magnesium: 0.61 mmol/L (normal range 0.7–1.0 mmol/L).
Chest X-ray: small bilateral pleural effusions.

Questions

1 What rhythm is shown on this rhythm strip?
2 What is the likely cause of this arrhythmia?
3 What treatment would be appropriate?

ECG analysis

Rate	230 bpm
Rhythm	Polymorphic ventricular tachycardia
QRS axis	Varying
P waves	Not visible
PR interval	–
QRS duration	Broad
T waves	Not visible
QTc interval	Not measureable on this rhythm strip (but was prolonged at 510 ms on admission 12-lead ECG)

Answers

1 Polymorphic ventricular tachycardia (VT), also known as torsades de pointes.

2 Polymorphic VT has a number of recognized causes (see Commentary) which prolong the QT interval and predispose to polymorphic VT. In this patient's case the likely aetiology is the patient's electrolyte abnormalities (hypokalaemia and hypomagnesaemia).

3 The electrolyte abnormalities need to be corrected. Standard adult life support protocols should be followed.

Commentary

● Polymorphic VT is also called torsades de pointes (twisting of the points), a descriptive term referring to the characteristic undulating pattern on the ECG, with a variation in the direction of the QRS axis. It is an uncommon arrhythmia but is important to recognize as it carries a risk of precipitating ventricular fibrillation.

● Polymorphic VT occurs in the setting of QT interval prolongation, which can be due to:

- hereditary long QT syndromes
- certain anti-arrhythmic drug treatments, such as Class Ia, Ic and III anti-arrhythmics (and also drug interactions).
- electrolyte abnormalities (hypokalaemia and hypomagnesaemia).

● Urgent assessment is warranted, with referral to a cardiologist if necessary. Any causative drugs need to be identified and withdrawn, and electrolyte abnormalities corrected.

● In an emergency, standard adult life support protocols should be followed. Polymorphic VT can be treated by giving magnesium (which is often effective even if the magnesium level is normal) and correcting any other electrolyte abnormalities. Any drugs that can prolong the QT interval should be withdrawn. Temporary pacing, which increases the heart rate and thereby shortens the QT interval, can be helpful. In the congenital long QT syndromes, left cervical sympathectomy can sometimes be indicated to interrupt the sympathetic supply to the heart. An implantable cardioverter defibrillator may be required if the patient is judged to be at high risk of sudden cardiac death.

Further reading

Making Sense of the ECG: Torsades de pointes (polymorphic VT), p 56; Is the QTc interval longer than 0.44s? p 207. Yap YG, Camm AJ. Drug induced QT prolongation and torsades de pointes. *Heart* 2003; **89**: 1363–72.

CASE 62

Clinical scenario

Female, aged 71 years.

Presenting complaint
No specific complaints.

History of presenting complaint
Patient had been diagnosed with complete heart block a few years ago when presented with dizziness and fatigue. Attended family doctor surgery for routine 'well woman' check and was concerned when ECG performed by practice nurse was shown to doctor.

Past medical history
Angina, hypertension, diabetes mellitus. Had experienced feeling weak and dizzy last year – fractured her hip following a fall but now fully independent again.

Examination
Pulse: 60 bpm, regular.
Blood pressure: 146/90.
JVP: not elevated.
Heart sounds: normal.
Chest auscultation: unremarkable.
Peripheral oedema: nil.

Investigations
FBC: Hb 10.5, WCC 3.9, platelets 145.
U&E: Na 133, K 4.8, urea 5.9, creatinine 129.
Chest X-ray: normal heart size, clear lung fields.
Echocardiogram: mild mitral regurgitation into mildly dilated left atrium. Left ventricular function mildly impaired (ejection fraction 51 per cent).

Questions

1 What does this ECG show?
2 What is the mechanism of this?
3 What are the likely causes?
4 What are the key issues in managing this patient?

ECG analysis

Rate	60 bpm
Rhythm	Atrial and ventricular sequential pacing
QRS axis	Left axis deviation (−61°)
P waves	None visible
PR interval	N/A
QRS duration	Prolonged (186 ms)
T waves	Normal
QTc interval	Normal (430 ms)

Answers

1 Despite there being no visible P waves, the rhythm is regular. A small pacing 'spike' is seen immediately before each wide QRS complex – this is a ventricular pacing spike. In addition, there is an additional pacing spike about 160 ms before each QRS complex – these are the pacemaker signals to the atria which trigger atrial systole. This is **atrioventricular sequential (or 'dual chamber') pacing.**

2 The atrial lead in the atrial appendage only generates an electrical impulse if the sinoatrial node fails to do so; here, no sinoatrial node activity is apparent, so every atrial impulse is pacemaker-activated, according to a preset rate. The ventricular lead only generates an electrical impulse if ventricular contraction does not occur within a fixed time period after the atria have been paced. Here, every ventricular contraction is also pacemaker activated. If intrinsic atrial and/or ventricular electrical activity is present, the pacemaker will stay in 'sense' mode.

3 The patient had episodes of collapse due to complete heart block. As the individual was very active and the ECG showed P waves, a dual chamber pacemaker was implanted. This restores the electrical connection between atrium and ventricle, ensuring that atrial and ventricular stimuli are coordinated, avoiding 'pacemaker syncope' – atrial contraction against an atrioventricular valve closed by ventricular contraction. Dual chamber pacing mimics the normal physiological action of the heart.

4 Pacemaker function needs checking a few weeks after implantation and at regular intervals thereafter. 'End of battery life' can be predicted to within a few weeks and unit replacement planned. If the patient needs surgery, both surgeon and anaesthetist need to be informed that a pacemaker has been implanted. The pacemaker should be checked before and after surgery. Diathermy can generate a high-energy field affecting pacemaker function – when it is used, it should be bipolar, with the 'active' electrode placed at least 15 cm from the pacemaker and the 'indifferent' electrode as remote as possible.

Commentary

● The symptoms of complete heart block, dizziness, lack of energy, breathlessness and syncope are usually relieved by a permanent pacemaker.

● The choice of pacemaker is important. Atrioventricular sequential pacing is preferred if there is any atrial activity, to avoid pacemaker syndrome.

● Pacemakers may be single chamber (pacing the atrium in AAI mode or the ventricle in VVI mode) or dual chamber (pacing both atrium and/or ventricle).

Further reading

Making Sense of the ECG: Pacemakers, p 222.

CASE 63

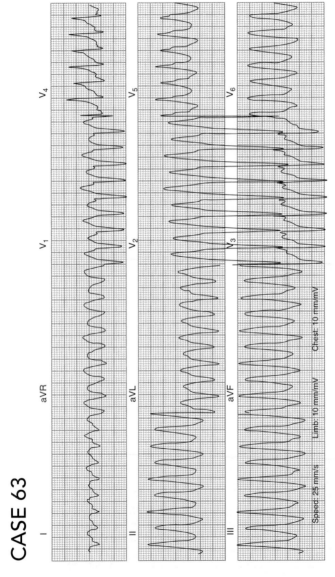

I, aVR, V1, V4, II, aVL, V2, V5, III, aVF, V3, V6

Speed: 25 mm/s   Limb: 10 mm/mV   Chest: 10 mm/mV

Figure adapted with permission from the BMJ Publishing Group (*Heart* 2000; **84**, 553–9).

Clinical scenario

Female, aged 27 years.

Presenting complaint
Palpitations.

History of presenting complaint
Intermittent episodes of rapid palpitations, particularly on heavy exertion.

Past medical history
No past medical history of note.

Examination
Pulse: 214 bpm, regular.
Blood pressure: 110/66.

JVP: not elevated.
Heart sounds: difficult to discern due to rapid tachycardia.
Chest auscultation: unremarkable.
No peripheral oedema.

Investigations
FBC: Hb 13.5, WCC 6.1, platelets 263.
U&E: Na 141, K 4.2, urea 4.8, creatinine 63.
Thyroid function: normal.
Chest X-ray: normal heart size, clear lung fields.
Echocardiogram (performed in sinus rhythm): normal cardiac structure and function.

Questions

1 Describe the appearances seen in this ECG.
2 What arrhythmia is shown on this ECG?
3 Where in the heart does this arrhythmia originate?
4 What is the prognosis in this condition?

ECG analysis

Rate	214 bpm
Rhythm	Ventricular tachycardia (idiopathic RVOT tachycardia)
QRS axis	Inferior
P waves	Not seen
PR interval	Not applicable
QRS duration	Broad complex
T waves	Abnormal
QTc interval	–

Additional comments

The QRS complexes in the chest leads show a left bundle branch block morphology.

Answers

1 This ECG shows a broad-complex tachycardia with a left bundle branch block appearance in the chest leads and an inferior QRS axis in the limb leads.

2 Ventricular tachycardia (VT).

3 This form of VT arises from the right ventricular outflow tract (RVOT), and is sometimes called idiopathic RVOT tachycardia. The origin of the arrhythmia in the RVOT is indicated by the left bundle branch block morphology and inferior QRS axis.

4 The prognosis for patients with *genuine* idiopathic ('structurally normal heart') RVOT tachycardia is thought to be good, with sudden death being rare. However, it is important not to misdiagnose idiopathic RVOT tachycardia by overlooking structural heart disease, in which case the prognosis is much worse. In particular, the VT seen in arrhythmogenic right ventricular cardiomyopathy (ARVC) can look similar to idiopathic RVOT tachycardia and careful cardiac imaging is therefore needed to distinguish between the two.

Commentary

● Monomorphic VT (where the QRS complexes look the same from beat to beat) arises from a specific area or 'focus' within the ventricles, as opposed to polymorphic VT (torsades de pointes) where the QRS complex morphology (and focus) changes constantly. VT arising from a specific focus may be amenable to treatment with ablation, and so identifying the location is important. The size of the focus is usually small in cases of idiopathic ('structurally normal heart') VT, making these forms of VT particularly suitable for ablation.

● Ventricular tachycardia in the structurally normal heart is relatively rare, accounting for approximately 10 per cent of cases of VT, and it usually arises in the RVOT (as in this example). Less commonly, idiopathic VT can arise in the left ventricle (idiopathic left ventricular verapamil-sensitive tachycardia).

● In the case of RVOT tachycardia, the left bundle branch block morphology indicates that the origin of the tachycardia is in the right ventricle (or the interventricular septum). The inferior QRS axis (indicated by the positive QRS complexes in the inferior leads: II, III and aVF) indicates that the focus lies superiorly in the ventricle. These two features together identify the RVOT as the location of the tachyarrhythmia.

● Pharmacological treatment options for idiopathic RVOT tachycardia include beta blockers (particularly when the arrhythmia is exercise related) or calcium channel blockers (verapamil or diltiazem – usually contraindicated in most other forms of VT). Ablation of the arrhythmogenic focus has a high success rate.

Further reading

Making Sense of the ECG: Ventricular tachycardia, p 53; How do I distinguish between VT and SVT? p 74.

Farzaneh-Far A, Lerman BB. Idiopathic ventricular outflow tract tachycardia. *Heart* 2005; **91**: 136–8.

Stevenson WG, Delacretaz, E. Radiofrequency catheter ablation of ventricular tachycardia. *Heart* 2000; **84**: 553–9.

CASE 64

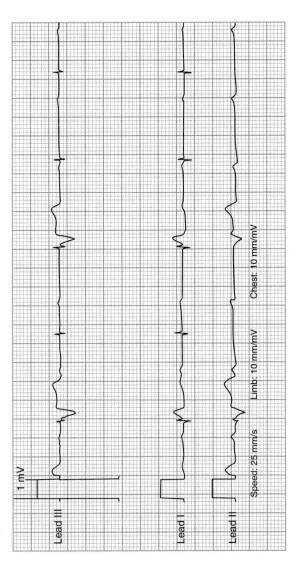

Lead III

Lead I

Lead II

1 mV

Speed: 25 mm/s   Limb: 10 mm/mV   Chest: 10 mm/mV

Clinical scenario

Male, aged 83 years.

Presenting complaint

Dizziness.

History of presenting complaint

Recently moved into sheltered accommodation to live near his daughter following his wife's death. Was found collapsed by warden. Seen in the emergency department and found to be extremely bradycardic. No further information available at time of admission.

Past medical history

Prescription in pocket – history of hypertension (on three anti-hypertensive agents). Permanent pacemaker implanted 11 years earlier.

Examination

Pulse: 33 bpm, irregular.
Blood pressure: 102/68.

JVP: normal.
Heart sounds: normal first and second sound; quiet ejection systolic murmur.
Chest auscultation: a few basal crackles.
No peripheral oedema.

Investigations

FBC: Hb 11.7, WCC 8.1, platelets 178.
U&E: Na 131, K 3.9, urea 12.3, creatinine 221.
Thyroid function: normal.
Troponin I: negative.
Chest X-ray: mild cardiomegaly, early pulmonary congestion.
Echocardiogram: thickened aortic valve with pressure gradient of 22 mmHg. Concentric left ventricular hypertrophy, systolic function mildly impaired (ejection fraction 44 per cent).

Questions

1 What does this ECG show?
2 What is the mechanism of this?
3 What are the key issues in managing this patient?

ECG analysis

Rate	<30 bpm
Rhythm	Pacing spikes with intermittent failure to capture
QRS axis	N/A
P waves	Present, with an atrial rate of 80 bpm
PR interval	N/A
QRS duration	Prolonged (132 ms)
T waves	N/A
QTc interval	N/A

Answers

1 This rhythm strip shows leads I, II and III. P waves can be seen (particularly clearly in lead II) with an atrial rate of around 80 bpm. There are also occasional pacing spikes, with a pacing rate of 66 bpm, but only two of these pacing spikes are followed by QRS complexes. A ventricular pacemaker is therefore trying to pace the ventricles at 66 bpm, but only intermittently succeeding in doing so. This is therefore underlying complete heart block and **ventricular (VVI) pacing with intermittent failure to capture.**

2 The pacing stimulus is delivered by the pacemaker but the ventricular myocardium fails to depolarize. This can be caused by:

- displacement of the ventricular lead from its optimal position adjacent to the ventricular myocardium
- malfunction of the pacing lead (e.g. lead fracture)
- a change in the pacing threshold (the voltage needed to depolarize the ventricle), as a result of myocardial infarction or ischaemia, electrolyte abnormalities or drug therapy
- inappropriate programming (inadequate voltage).

3 The underlying cause of the loss of capture needs to be identified and addressed (see above). A chest X-ray will show the position of the pacing lead and whether it has become dislodged. If the problem is due to a problem with the pacemaker system itself, it may require reprogramming, or repositioning/replacement of the pacing lead.

Commentary

● Pacemaker problems include failures in sensing and failures in pacing.

● **Failure to sense**: the intrinsic intra-cardiac activity is not recognized by the pacemaker because of:

- inappropriate lead placement
- lead displacement – usually within a few weeks of pacemaker installation
- lead fracture or insulation defect – can occur months or years after installation; manufacturer will advise if problem occurs with a faulty batch; advise manufacturer if lead fracture identified. Occasionally due to 'twiddler's syndrome' (tendency for patient to rotate the pacemaker unit itself – avoidable by ensuring the size of the pacemaker's pocket is minimized during wound closure)
- connector problem – lead connection to pacemaker poor
- inappropriate programming
- component failure, e.g. magnetic reed switch jammed (rare).

● **Failure to pace**: a pacing stimulus is not delivered when expected, or a stimulus is delivered but the myocardium does not depolarize. A stimulus will not be delivered with:

- connector problem – a ratchet screwdriver with preset torque ensures satisfactory attachment of the lead to the pacemaker unit. More of a problem if an 'old style' lead is connected to a 'modern' pacemaker unit
- lead fracture – this is rare but will trigger a manufacturer's alert
- pulse generator failure – pacemaker failure is usually due to battery depletion.

● **Oversensing**: Pacemaker detects signals other than those intended (e.g. 'cross talk' between atrial and ventricular components of dual chamber pacemaker); this can usually be electrically 'tuned out' by the cardiac physiologist.

● Lead displacement may occur:

- early (within 6 weeks) – about 1 per cent of ventricular leads and 4 per cent of atrial leads get displaced
- late – usually affecting the atrial lead.

Further reading

Making Sense of the ECG: Pacemakers, p 222.

CASE 65

Speed: 25 mm/s   Limb: 10 mm/mV   Chest: 10 mm/mV

Clinical scenario

Female, aged 72 years.

Presenting complaint

Exertional breathlessness. Orthopnoea.

History of presenting complaint

One-year history of gradually worsening breathlessness with a reduction in exercise capacity – the patient can now walk 100 m on level ground. Recent orthopnoea – the patient sleeps with four pillows.

Past medical history

Inferior myocardial infarction 7 years ago.
Anteroseptal myocardial infarction 4 years ago.
Essential tremor.

Examination

Resting tremor affecting the hands.
Pulse: 90 bpm, regular.

Blood pressure: 118/74.
JVP: elevated by 3 cm.
Heart sounds: soft (2/6) pan-systolic murmur at apex.
Chest auscultation: bibasal inspiratory crackles.
No peripheral oedema.

Investigations

FBC: Hb 11.8, WCC 5.9, platelets 240.
U&E: Na 137, K 4.1, urea 7.7, creatinine 118.
Chest X-ray: moderate cardiomegaly, pulmonary oedema.
Echocardiogram: dilated left ventricle with moderately impaired systolic function (ejection fraction 35 per cent). Mild functional mitral regurgitation.

Questions

1 What heart rhythm is evident on this ECG?
2 Are there any other ECG findings?
3 What are the likely causes of these findings?

ECG analysis

Rate	90 bpm
Rhythm	Sinus rhythm
QRS axis	Normal (−56°)
P waves	Normal
PR interval	Prolonged (205 ms)
QRS duration	Normal (78 ms)
T waves	Normal
QTc interval	Normal (442 ms)

Additional comments

There are inferior Q waves and there is poor R wave progression in leads V_1–V_5.

Answers

1 Sinus rhythm, which is best appreciated in the chest leads (V_1–V_6).

2 There are several findings:

• The baseline in the limb leads is erratic and masks the P waves, making it difficult to discern the underlying rhythm in these leads. The rhythm is seen much more clearly in the chest leads.

• There are inferior Q waves.

• There is poor anterior R wave progression (affecting leads V_1–V_5).

• There is left axis deviation.

• There is mild first-degree atrioventricular block (PR interval 205 ms).

3 There are two causes.

• The erratic baseline is a consequence of the essential tremor, producing musculoskeletal artefact on the ECG recording.

• Ischaemic heart disease would account for the inferior Q waves (old inferior myocardial infarction), poor anterior R wave progression (old anteroseptal myocardial infarction), left axis deviation (which can be a consequence of inferior myocardial infarction) and mild impairment of atrioventricular conduction.

Commentary

● The ECG records the electrical activity of the heart, but this is not the only source of electrical activity in the body. Skeletal muscle activity is also picked up on the ECG.

● Where possible, patients should lie still during an ECG recording to minimize skeletal muscle artefact, but this is not always possible, particularly if the patient:

- is uncooperative or agitated
- is in respiratory distress
- has a movement disorder.

● The presence of electrical artefact which is much more marked in the limb leads than in the chest leads (as in this example) strongly suggests that skeletal muscle interference from limb movement is the cause.

● The use of signal-averaged ECGs (to 'average out' random electrical artefacts by combining a number of PQRST complexes) can help to reduce the impact of skeletal muscle artefact, particularly during exercise treadmill testing. However, signal-averaged recordings can introduce artefactual changes of their own and such recordings should therefore always be interpreted with discretion.

Further reading

Making Sense of the ECG: How do I record an ECG? p 16; Patient movement, p 220.

CASE 66

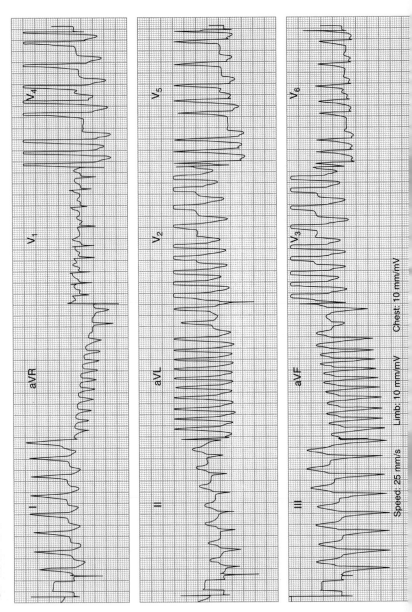

Speed: 25 mm/s   Limb: 10 mm/mV   Chest: 10 mm/mV

Clinical scenario

Female, aged 58 years.

Presenting complaint
Palpitations of sudden onset.

History of presenting complaint
Woken from sleep with racing heart beat and breathlessness.

Past medical history
Nil significant.

Examination
Pulse: 228 bpm, irregularly irregular.
Blood pressure: 110/50.
JVP: not visible.
Heart sounds: hard to assess (tachycardia).
Chest auscultation: fine basal crackles.
No peripheral oedema.

Investigations
FBC: Hb 13.9, WCC 8.1, platelets 233.
U&E: Na 137, K 4.2, urea 5.3, creatinine 88.
Thyroid function: normal.
Troponin I: negative.
Chest X-ray: mild cardiomegaly, early pulmonary congestion.

Questions

1 What does this ECG show?
2 What is the mechanism of this?
3 What are the key issues in managing this patient?

ECG analysis

Rate	228 bpm
Rhythm	Atrial fibrillation with ventricular pre-excitation
QRS axis	Left axis deviation (−49°)
P waves	Not visible
PR interval	N/A
QRS duration	Prolonged (130 ms)
T waves	Inverted in anterolateral leads
QTc interval	Difficult to assess at such high heart rates

Answers

1 This ECG shows irregularly irregular QRS complexes with no discernible P waves, the hallmark of atrial fibrillation. The ventricular rate is very fast. The QRS complexes are somewhat broad and have an odd morphology, not typical of a left or right bundle branch block. This is **atrial fibrillation with ventricular pre-excitation** in Wolff–Parkinson–White (WPW) syndrome.

2 Conduction from atria to ventricles is usually through a single connection involving the atrioventricular node and bundle of His. The ventricles are normally protected from rapid atrial activity by the refractory period of the atrioventricular node. In WPW syndrome, there is an additional *accessory pathway* which conducts electrical activity to the ventricles at a faster rate than the atrioventricular node. If atrial fibrillation develops, most impulses will be conducted via the accessory pathway, so high ventricular rates can be achieved. These beats will contain delta waves as a result of ventricular pre-excitation (see Case 16). Some impulses will be conducted normally via the atrioventricular node and so normal QRS complexes may be visible at intervals.

3 At very fast heart rates there is a risk of ventricular fibrillation, so an urgent cardioversion should be considered. Alternatively, you can use a drug that slows conduction through the accessory pathway such as amiodarone or flecainide.

Commentary

● Atrial fibrillation in WPW syndrome can resemble ventricular tachycardia, but AF is irregular whereas ventricular tachycardia is regular.

● In WPW syndrome with atrial fibrillation, the ventricular rate can be very fast due to conduction via the accessory pathway. Blocking the atrioventricular node can paradoxically increase the heart rate even more, by directing all the impulses down the accessory pathway, precipitating ventricular fibrillation. Drugs such as adenosine, beta blockers, verapamil and digoxin must therefore be *avoided* in these patients.

● Urgent cardioversion is the preferred treatment, especially if the patient is hypotensive or in heart failure.

● Patients with WPW syndrome who have had an episode of atrial fibrillation should be referred to a cardiac electrophysiologist for consideration of an accessory pathway ablation procedure.

Further reading

Making Sense of the ECG: Wolff–Parkinson–White syndrome, p 114; Atrial fibrillation in Wolff–Parkinson–White syndrome, p 52.

CASE 67

Speed: 25 mm/s   Limb: 10 mm/mV   Chest: 10 mm/mV

Clinical scenario

Male, aged 73 years.

Presenting complaint
Breathlessness and peripheral oedema.

History of presenting complaint
Three month history of progressive breathlessness and peripheral oedema, with a steady fall in exercise capacity.

Past medical history
Multiple myeloma.

Examination
Patient comfortable at rest but breathless on exertion.
Pulse: 78 bpm, regular.

Blood pressure: 118/78.
JVP: elevated.
Heart sounds: normal.
Chest auscultation: bilateral inspiratory crackles.
Moderate peripheral oedema.

Investigations
FBC: Hb 10.8, WCC 8.3, platelets 174.
U&E: Na 139, K 4.5, urea 8.2, creatinine 141.
Chest X-ray: pulmonary oedema.
Echocardiogram: moderate hypertrophy of left and right ventricles, with an echogenic 'granular' appearance of myocardium, and evidence of diastolic dysfunction ('stiff ventricles'). Dilatation of left and right atria.

Questions

1 What abnormalities are seen on this ECG?
2 How do these abnormalities relate to the echocardiographic findings?
3 What is the likely clinical diagnosis?

ECG analysis

Rate	78 bpm
Rhythm	Sinus rhythm
QRS axis	Normal ($+30°$)
P waves	Normal
PR interval	Borderline short (110 ms)
QRS duration	Normal (90 ms)
T waves	Widespread inversion
QTc interval	Mildly prolonged (456 ms)

Additional comments

There is a dominant R wave in lead V_1, and tall R waves in leads V_3–V_5.

Answers

1 This ECG contains several abnormalities. The main ones are:

- dominant R waves in the right precordial leads
- tall R waves in leads V_3–V_5

- ST depression and T wave inversion in the anterolateral leads
- T wave inversion in leads II and aVF

2 The dominant R waves in the right precordial leads are consistent with right ventricular hypertrophy. The tall R waves in leads V_3–V_5 are consistent with left ventricular hypertrophy, and the ST segment and T wave abnormalities are consistent with ventricular 'strain' in association with the hypertrophy. The echocardiogram supports these findings, revealing moderate hypertrophy of left and right ventricles.

3 The presence of moderate left and right ventricular hypertrophy with an echogenic 'granular' appearance, together with dilatation of both atria, in the context of a patient with multiple myeloma, is suggestive of cardiac amyloidosis secondary to light chain amyloidosis. This diagnosis can be confirmed by cardiac biopsy.

Commentary

● Right ventricular hypertrophy causes a 'dominant' R wave (i.e. bigger than the S wave) in the leads that 'look at' the right ventricle, particularly V_1. Right ventricular hypertrophy can also cause:

- right axis deviation
- deep S waves in leads V_5 and V_6
- right bundle branch block (RBBB)
- ST depression and/or T wave inversion in the right precordial leads (when severe).

● Right ventricular hypertrophy is not the only cause of a positive R wave in lead V_1. Other causes include:

- posterior myocardial infarction
- Wolff–Parkinson–White syndrome Type A (left-sided accessory pathway)
- dextrocardia.

● Causes of right ventricular hypertrophy include pressure overload on the right ventricle (e.g. pulmonary stenosis, pulmonary hypertension) or hypertrophic cardiomyopathies affecting the right ventricular myocardium. The treatment of right ventricular hypertrophy is that of the underlying cause.

● In this case the right (and left) ventricular hypertrophy are the result of cardiac amyloidosis, the deposition of amyloid protein in the myocardium. Cardiac amyloidosis most commonly occurs in multiple myeloma (as in this case) and results in stiffening of the ventricles (diastolic dysfunction), leading to a restrictive cardiomyopathy and the clinical features of congestive cardiac failure. It can also cause conduction disturbances and arrhythmias.

Further reading

Making Sense of the ECG: Left ventricular hypertrophy, p 136; Right ventricular hypertrophy, p 139.

Selvanayagam JB, Hawkins PN, Paul B, *et al.* Evaluation and management of the cardiac amyloidosis. *J Am Coll Cardiol* 2007; **50**: 2101–10.

CASE 68

Figure adapted with permission from the BMJ Publishing Group (*Heart* 2006; **92**: 559–68).

Clinical scenario

Male, aged 35 years.

Presenting complaint
Found collapsed at work.

History of presenting complaint
Reported feeling unwell but insisted on staying at desk.
Collapsed and was given immediate basic life support.
When the paramedics arrived, he was in ventricular
fibrillation and had two DC shocks.

Past medical history
Had always been fit and well. Keen marathon runner.

Examination
Pulse: 60 bpm, regular.
Blood pressure: 134/84.

JVP: not elevated.
Heart sounds: normal.
Chest auscultation: unremarkable.
No peripheral oedema.

Investigations
FBC: Hb 16.7, WCC 6.7, platelets 265.
U&E: Na 140, K 4.3, urea 4.0, creatinine 97.
Troponin I: negative.
Chest X-ray: normal heart size, clear lung fields.
Echocardiogram: normal aortic and mitral valves. Left
ventricular function good (ejection fraction 65 per cent).

Questions

1 What does this ECG show?
2 What is the likely cause of the collapse?
3 What is the underlying mechanism?
4 What are the key issues in managing this patient?

ECG analysis

Rate	60 bpm
Rhythm	Sinus rhythm
QRS axis	Normal (+54°)
P waves	Normal
PR interval	Normal (190 ms)
QRS duration	Normal (120 ms)
T waves	Normal
QTc interval	Normal (360 ms)

Additional comments

There is ST segment elevation in leads V_1–V_3 and a right bundle branch block morphology.

Answers

1 There is ST segment elevation in the right chest leads (V_1–V_3) and a right bundle branch block (RBBB) morphology – this combination of ECG signs is suggestive of **Brugada syndrome.**

2 In patients with a structurally normal heart but with the ECG characteristics shown above, Brugada syndrome is associated with syncopal or sudden death episodes. Collapse may be due to fast, polymorphic ventricular tachycardia or ventricular fibrillation, usually occurring without warning.

3 Inheritance is autosomal dominant in around 50 per cent of cases and there is an 8:1 male:female ratio. Abnormalities have been identified in the genes coding for ion channels, and in particular the sodium channel gene *SCN5A*.

4 The diagnosis of Brugada syndrome can be difficult as the ECG changes above may be intermittent or their significance overlooked. ECG abnormalities may be 'unmasked' pharmacologically with flecainide, procainamide or ajmaline. It is important to exclude electrolyte disorders (hyperkalaemia and hypercalcaemia), and structural heart disease. No drug has been proven effective at preventing arrhythmias or reducing mortality in sudden cardiac death (SCD) survivors, and so there is a low threshold for using an implantable cardioverter-fibrillator (ICD).

Commentary

- Epidemiology:
  - 60 per cent of patients with aborted SCD with typical Brugada ECG have a family history of sudden death or a family with similar ECGs.
  - Brugada syndrome probably accounts for about half of all cases of idiopathic ventricular fibrillation.
  - Incidence probably underestimated: incidence varies with population — 26–38/100 000 per year in South East Asia.
  - Recognized worldwide but greatest prevalence in the Far East: 1:2000 of adult Japanese; 1:30 000 in Belgium.
  - Most common cause of sudden death in South Asians under 50 with apparently structurally normal heart.
  - 40 per cent with typical ECG will have a first episode of ventricular tachycardia or sudden death in 3 years, unless asymptomatic with abnormal ECG after drugs.
- Prognosis:
  - After syncope or aborted sudden death, 30 per cent have new episode of polymorphic ventricular tachycardia within 2 years.

- 30 per cent of asymptomatic patients with typical ECG have first polymorphic ventricular tachycardia or ventricular fibrillation within 2 years.
- ICD prevents sudden death in *symptomatic* individuals whether ECG normalizes or not.
- ICD is also beneficial in *asymptomatic* individuals if spontaneously abnormal ECG and inducible ventricular tachycardia/ventricular fibrillation.
- Anti-arrhythmic drugs do not protect and the role of an ICD is not clear if the patient is asymptomatic with an abnormal ECG but ventricular tachycardia/ventricular fibrillation is not inducible.

Further reading

Making Sense of the ECG: Are the ST segments elevated? p 159; Brugada syndrome, p 176.
Fitzpatrick AP, Cooper P. Diagnosis and management of patients with blackouts. *Heart* 2006; **92**: 559–68.
Web resource: Brugada Syndrome (www.brugada.org).

CASE 69

Speed: 25 mm/s   Limb: 10 mm/mV   Chest: 10 mm/mV

Clinical scenario

Male, aged 28 years.

Presenting complaint

Palpitations.

History of presenting complaint

Four-month history of episodic palpitations – sudden onset rapid heartbeat, lasting up to 15 min, followed by sudden termination of palpitations. The patient was asymptomatic during the recording of this ECG rhythm strip.

Past medical history

Nil.

Examination

Pulse: 54 bpm, regular.
Blood pressure: 136/88.
JVP: not elevated.
Heart sounds: normal.
Chest auscultation: unremarkable.
No peripheral oedema.

Investigations

FBC: Hb 14.7, WCC 5.8, platelets 339.
U&E: Na 142, K 5.1, urea 4.5, creatinine 76.
Thyroid function: normal.

Questions

1 This rhythm strip is taken from a 24-h ambulatory ECG recording – what does it show?
2 What can cause this?
3 What would you do next?

ECG analysis

Rate	Difficult to assess in view of bizarre rhythm
Rhythm	Bizarre – there appear to be two distinct overlapping rhythms
QRS axis	Unable to assess (single lead)
P waves	Difficult to assess in view of bizarre rhythm
PR interval	Difficult to assess in view of bizarre rhythm
QRS duration	Difficult to assess in view of bizarre rhythm
T waves	Difficult to assess in view of bizarre rhythm
QTc interval	Difficult to assess in view of bizarre rhythm

Answers

1 This is a very odd ECG recording. On close inspection there appear to be two distinct heart rhythms occurring simultaneously, with no obvious correlation between them. In some cases two distinct QRS complexes occur on top of, or close to, each other.

2 In this case, the rhythm strip was made using an old 24-h ECG recorder that used cassette tapes to record the ECG. The cassette tape had been accidentally re-used without the previous recording having been deleted, and so two recordings from different patients ended up on the same cassette tape. When the tape was analyzed, the two recordings appeared simultaneously on one rhythm strip. A similar appearance can be seen in patients who have received a heterotopic 'piggy-back' heart transplant, in which a donor heart is connected to the patient's own heart. Both hearts operate independently, and so an ECG will show two distinct heart rhythms, one from each heart.

3 This recording should be discarded and a new 24-h ECG recording should be made.

Commentary

● Always consider the possibility of artefact in 'bizarre' ECGs, particularly when they do not correlate with what you know about the patient's clinical details.

● It is very unusual for ambulatory ECG recordings from two different patients to be recorded onto a single cassette tape in such a way that both recordings can still be detected by the computer software when the tape is analysed. Rare errors of this kind highlight the importance of taking a careful and structured approach to ECG interpretation, and to ensure that any abnormalities you see can be accounted for.

● This kind of recording error should no longer be possible now that cassette tapes have been superseded by solid-state digital recording technology in ambulatory ECG monitoring.

● In patients with a heterotopic 'piggy-back' heart transplant, a similar 'double ECG' can be seen. In this type of heart transplant, the recipient's heart is left in situ to supplement the function of the donor heart. Heterotopic heart transplants are rarely performed, but may be appropriate if the donor heart is unable to function alone (for example, if the recipient's body size is much greater than that of the donor's, or if the recipient has pulmonary hypertension).

Further reading

Making Sense of the ECG: Artefacts on the ECG, p 217.

CASE 70

Speed: 25 mm/s   Limb: 10 mm/mV   Chest: 10 mm/mV

Clinical scenario

Male, aged 36 years.

Presenting complaint
Breathlessness on exertion.

History of presenting complaint
Patient was fit and well until 12 months earlier. Heart failure had developed after a flu-like illness – viral myocarditis diagnosed. Assessed for cardiac transplant but turned down as had had problems with depression including one (much regretted) suicide attempt. An alternative operation had been offered and performed, and this ECG was recorded post-surgery.

Past medical history
Viral myocarditis.
Depression.

Examination
Pulse: 96 bpm, regular.
Blood pressure: 108/76.

JVP: not elevated.
Heart sounds: normal.
Chest auscultation: unremarkable.
No peripheral oedema.

Investigations
FBC: Hb 15.9, WCC 6.6, platelets 222.
U&E: Na 143, K 4.1, urea 4.7, creatinine 106.
Thyroid function: normal.
Troponin I: negative.
Chest X-ray: mild cardiomegaly, early pulmonary congestion.
Echocardiogram: moderate mitral regurgitation and dilated left atrium. Left ventricular function severely impaired (ejection fraction 23 per cent).

Questions

1 What does this ECG show?
2 What operation has this patient undergone?

ECG analysis

Rate	96 bpm
Rhythm	Sinus rhythm
QRS axis	Normal (+23°)
P waves	Normal
PR interval	Normal (184 ms)
QRS duration	Normal (110 ms)
T waves	Inverted in inferior and anterolateral leads
QTc interval	Normal (440 ms)

Additional comments

After some of the QRS complexes there is a pacing spike followed by a burst of electrical 'noise' from skeletal muscle.

Answers

1 The ECG shows a normal P wave, PR interval and QRS duration and multiple pacing spikes which occur after many of the QRS complexes. This is the ECG from a patient who has undergone a **dynamic cardiomyoplasty**.

2 This operation involves mobilizing the patient's left latissimus dorsi muscle as a pedicle graft, wrapping the free end around the heart and stimulating it to contract in synchrony with cardiac systole. Based on animal and human studies, the benefits of this operation are believed to be due to:

- a chronic girdling effect due to the wrapping of latissimus dorsi around the heart, resulting in stabilization of the ventricular remodelling process and a decrease in left ventricular dilatation
- active systolic assistance to decrease myocardial stress.

The operation is performed for patients with New York Heart Association (NYHA) class III heart failure which is symptomatic despite maximal medical treatment but who still have some cardiac reserve. The skeletal muscle must be 'trained' to work like cardiac muscle – a pacing electrode is placed within the muscle and over a period of weeks stimulated by an impulse generator synchronized with cardiac contraction.

Commentary

● Dynamic cardiomyoplasty has been used as an alternative to cardiac transplantation.

● Perioperative mortality is about 10 per cent.

● 'Muscle transformation' – training the latissimus dorsi muscle by pacing every fourth, third, alternate and finally every cardiac contraction – takes at least eight weeks.

● Cardiac augmentation has been disappointing, although there may be a subjective improvement in symptoms.

● Trials report an increase in left ventricular ejection fraction, left ventricular stroke index and stroke work.

● Outcomes have been disappointing and the operation abandoned in the USA and UK.

● Benefits in patients with Chagas' disease have been more encouraging, probably because the myocardium is not thinned and poorly contractile (as compared with ischaemic cardiomyopathy).

Further reading

Treasure T. Cardiac myoplasty with the latissimus dorsi muscle. *Lancet* 1991; **337**: 1383–4.

Yilmaz MB, Tufekcioglu O, Korkmaz S *et al.* Dynamic cardiomyoplasty: impact of effective pacing. *Int J Cardiol* 2003; **91**: 101–2.

Index

and left bundle branch block   32
myocarditis
  coexistent   181
  viral   176–7, 278–81
myocardium, enhanced automaticity   224
myomectomy, septal   240

nicotine   13
nitrates   201
'noise'   280
non-shockable rhythms   108–9
non-ST segment elevation acute coronary
        syndrome (NSTEACS)   49
  inferolateral   66–9
  treatment   68
non-ST segment elevation myocardial infarction
        (NSTEMI)   49
  inferolateral   66–9
normal values   xv, 196
nuclear myocardial perfusion   32
nucleus ambiguus   8

oedema, peripheral   267
opiates   48
'Osborn wave'   164–5

'P mitrale'   84–5
P wave   133
  absent   24, 60, 61, 96, 104, 148
  and atrial ectopic beats   12, 13
  broad, bifid   84–5
  focused away from the sinoatrial node   120
  hidden   117
  inverted   37, 77, 148, 156
  missed   56
  small   117
  variable interval   152, 153
pacemaker syndrome   144, 248, 249
pacemakers
  AAI   145, 152
  AAIR   145, 188–9
  DDD   144, 145, 152
  DDDR   145, 192
  dual chamber   144, 145, 152, 188–9, 246–9
  failure to pace   257
  failure to sense   257
  functional checks on   248
  lead placement problems   256–7
  oversensing   257
  pacing codes   145, 188, 189
  permanent   188–9, 192

  problems with   254–7
  reprogramming/repositioning   256
  single chamber   144, 145, 152, 188–9,
        249
  for sinus arrest   152
  ventricular pacing with intermittent failure to
        capture   254–7
  VVI   144, 145
  VVIR   145
pacemakers of the heart
  bundle   133, 193
  subsidiary   133, 193
pacing   132, 133
  atrial   186–9, 248
  atrioventricular sequential (dual chamber)
        246–9
  permanent   188–9, 192
    for bradycardia   21
    for complete heart block   142–5
    and second-degree atrioventricular block
        88, 89
    for sinoatrial node exit block   80
  temporary
    for bradycardia   21
    for polymorphic ventricular tachycardia
        245
    and second-degree atrioventricular block
        88
    for third-degree atrioventricular block
        133, 193
  ventricular   142–5, 248, 254–7
pacing 'spikes'   188
  atrial   248
  ventricular   248, 256
pain see chest pain
pain relief   48
palpitations   10–13, 22–5, 34–41, 57, 65,
        86–9, 134–7, 234–41, 250–3
  episodic   122–5, 274–7
  rapid regular   74–7, 114–17, 146–9
  of sudden onset   262–5
paper speed   210–13
percutaneous coronary intervention (PCI)   48,
        128
  primary   28–9, 49, 112–13, 160, 208
  'rescue'   29, 113
pericardial effusion   181
pericarditis   178–81
  causes   180
  testing for   180
perioperative events   129, 133
post-cardiac arrest   218–21